10 Habits That Mess Up a Woman's Diet

Simple Strategies to Eat Right, Lose Weight & Reclaim Your Health

WITHDRAWN

Elizabeth Somer, M.A., R.D.

McGraw-Hill

New York   Chicago   San Francisco   Lisbon   London   Madrid   Mexico City
Milan   New Delhi   San Juan   Seoul   Singapore   Sydney   Toronto

Library of Congress Cataloging-in-Publication Data

Somer, Elizabeth.
    10 habits that mess up a woman's diet : simple strategies to eat right, lose weight, and reclaim your health / Elizabeth Somer.
        p.   cm.
    Includes bibliographical references and index.
    ISBN 0-07-146228-7 (alk. paper)
    1. Weight loss.   2. Women—Health and hygiene.   I. Title: Ten habits that mess up a woman's diet.   II. Title.

    RM222.2.S6545   2006
    613'.04244—dc22   2005013469

    3 4 5 6 7 8 9 0   FGR/FGR   0 9 8 7 6

ISBN 0-07-146228-7

McGraw-Hill books are available at special quantity discounts to use as premiums and sales promotions, or for use in corporate training programs. For more information, please write to the Director of Special Sales, Professional Publishing, McGraw-Hill, Two Penn Plaza, New York, NY 10121-2298. Or contact your local bookstore.

The nutritional and health information presented in this book is based on an in-depth review of the current scientific literature. It is intended only as a resource guide to help you make informed decisions; it is not meant to replace the advice of a physician or therapist, or to serve as a guide to self-treatment. Always seek competent medical help for any health condition or if there is any question about the appropriateness of a procedure or health recommendation.

This book is printed on acid-free paper.

To my children, two sisters, best friends, nieces, and girlfriends, and the men who love them. I am grateful every day for having them in my life.

Contents

Preface   ix
Acknowledgments   xiii

Introduction: The Scoop on Women's Diets   1
The Hourglass Diet   2
We're Eating Too Much   2
We're Not Eating Enough   4
Get a Real Food Life: The Six Preplanning Steps
    to Eating Well   8
What Does Healthy Eating Look Like?   14
The Ultimate Diet Plan   15
Those 10 Habits   19

Habit 1: Mindless Eating   25
Invisible Calories   26
Eating on Autopilot: The Downside   29
Nibbling Is OK   31
Mindful Breakfasts   36
Kick the Habit   40
Choose a New Habit   44
Mindful Eating   47

Habit 2: Putting Others' Needs Ahead of Our Own   51
Love 'n' Marriage: Together in Eating   52
Babies and Weight Gain   56
Mealtime Peer Pressure   57
Dining Out Can Do Us In   58
Kick the Habit   60
Keep Your Diet in Perspective   71

Habit 3: Not Being Honest   75
Fessing Up Is Hard to Do   78
Portion Distortion   82

Kick the Habit   89
How Much Exercise Is Enough?   94
It's Within Your Grasp   97

Habit 4: Skip the Broccoli, Eat the Fries   101
Nothing Is Better for You than Produce   103
How Much Are You Eating?   105
Which Ones Are the Best?   110
Produce to Avoid   114
Kick the Habit   116
Ya Gotta Love 'em   124

Habit 5: Setting Off Without a Plan   125
Kick the Habit   127
Outside the Box   133
Two "Must-Have" Habits   134
Practice, Practice, Practice   136
The Only Way to Get Better Is to Change   136

Habit 6: Excuses, Excuses, Excuses   149
You Can Change   150
Kick the Habit   151
Take Responsibility   166

Habit 7: I'm Moody—Let's Eat!   167
Food for Solace or Sustenance?   169
Food and Mood   170
Dieting = Weight Gain   176
Kick the Habit   178
Your Mood Is More than Just Diet   190

Habit 8: Give Me the Quick Fix, Now!   191
Tell Me Again Why Diets Don't Work   193
Diet Myths Debunked   196
Kick the Habit   203
Commit to Health   215

Habit 9: Drinking Away Our Waistlines   **217**

Silent Calories   217
Cola Calories   218
Josephine Six-Pack   220
The Dark Side of Alcohol   224
Kick the Habit   226
Think Moderation   233

Habit 10: The All-or-Nothing Approach to Dieting   **235**

Why the All-or-Nothing Mentality Fails   236
All-or-Nothing and Your Weight   237
Self-Talk: The Chatter Inside Your Head   238
Kick the Habit   239
Give Yourself Some Slack   251

Simple Steps, Big Results   **253**

The Salami Principle: Simple Steps   256
The Ultimate Goal   261

Selected Reading   269
References   271
Index   301

Preface

Are you at your wit's end when it comes to your weight or your health?

Are you frustrated and mad at yourself for having tried one diet after another, only to lose weight initially by nibbling on fat-free celery and rice cakes or low-carb eggs and bacon, but then gain it all back, and then some?

Do you ever wonder why you eat the same foods as your best friends, yet your friends are thin and healthy, and you're not?

Do you doubt you have the willpower to stick with a healthy eating plan?

Have you ever considered just giving up and living with the gradual weight gain that seems to be your lot in life?

If so, you must be a card-carrying member of the distinguished group called—*Women*. Just about every woman, at one time or another, has tried and failed to eat better or lose weight. Dieting is our pastime, our nemesis, and our obsession. Yet, despite decades of dieting, hundreds of different diets, and a billion weight-loss attempts, women in the developed world are heavier than ever. Even though women in the United States diet more vigorously, take better care of their health, and, in general, eat better than men, almost 7 out of every 10 are overweight, and more than 3 in 10 are obese—and the numbers increase with each passing year. Obesity experts predict that unless this trend is stopped, almost all women will be overweight by the year 2050! What's up with that?!

10 Habits That Do Us In

Maybe worrying constantly about what we are eating, switching from low-carb to fat-free and then back to low-carb, and collecting bottles of weight-loss pills, potions, and powders isn't the solution. I'll bet my nutrition credentials that the real reason why you haven't lost that excess weight—be it 5, 50, or 150 pounds—has more to do with a habit or two that you unconsciously practice every day. You're probably not even aware of how that habit is undermining your best efforts to be the lean, healthy, energetic, gorgeous woman you were born to be.

I know these habits intimately. There are 10 of them. When I haven't caved in to them myself, I've helped women for the past 25 years recognize and fix one or more of these little habits so that they finally lost the weight or saw the numbers drop on their lab reports. Take Laura, for example, who swore to me that she didn't eat anything but vegetables, yet later realized that she ate hundreds of extra calories every day by grazing on leftover PB&J sandwiches, mac and cheese, and chips as she cleaned up after her kids (see Habit 1: Mindless Eating). Another client couldn't lose weight despite her best efforts, until she finally admitted that she hadn't been completely truthful to herself or to me about how much she exercised (see Habit 3: Not Being Honest). Sally had tried a variety of get-thin-fast diets, only to permanently lose weight when she stopped dieting and started taking good care of herself (see Habit 8: Give Me the Quick Fix, Now!). Then there was Nancy, who had no idea that her favorite drink, a martini with an olive, packed the calorie equivalent of a slice of pizza; on top of her total food intake for the day, it was just enough extra calories to keep her from losing the last 5 pounds (see Habit 9: Drinking Away Our Waistlines).

If you have any doubts that one or more of these or other habits might be getting in your way of feeling and looking great, take a minute and answer "yes" or "no" to these questions:

— Have you ever nibbled off of a partner's plate, taste-tested while cooking, taken a fork to an entire cake, or eaten anything straight from the container while standing at the kitchen counter?
— Do you have trouble resisting second or third helpings at parties or buffets?
— Have you ever finished a too-big plate of food at a restaurant, felt uncomfortably full, and wondered why you ate the whole thing?

— Does the thought that you should include at least eight fruits and vegetables in your daily diet seem overwhelming?

— Do you ever skip meals, eat haphazardly, or fall short of your goal to "eat better"?

— Have you ever heard yourself say, "I don't have time to exercise" or "I've tried dieting, but I just can't seem to keep the weight off"?

— Are you likely to drown your sorrows or stress in a bag of chips or a pint of ice cream?

— Have you tried more than one type of diet, such as low-carb, food-combining, or a soup diet, in the past year?

— Do you drink more than seven soft drink or alcoholic beverages a week, or more than one a day?

— Do you consider yourself either "on" or "off" a diet?

Whether you answered "yes" to one or all of the above, you're no stranger to the habits that block many women's chances of ever seeing their dream number on the scale or a perfect-health report from the doctor.

You're not alone. Almost every one of us does it. We say we want to be lean and sexy, eat so our skin glows and our hair shines, exercise so we will look and feel younger, have more energy, and improve our diets to lower our risk for diseases, such as heart disease, diabetes, or cancer. We try one diet after another, fail repeatedly, and blame the whole mess on our lack of willpower, sluggish metabolism, or fate. Yet, the real reason is a habit or two that is secretly ruining our efforts. These 10 habits are subtle. They often are second nature, so we don't even know we are taking one step backward for every step forward, serving as our own worst enemy when it comes to reaching our health and weight goals.

Tough Love, Healthy Bodies

Every women needs a best friend to tell her the truth, no matter what—someone who will let her know just before she makes her grand entrance, ready to wow the crowd, that she has a stream of toilet paper trailing from her panty hose. That's what *10 Habits*

That Mess Up a Woman's Diet is all about. This book is like your best friend, the one who honestly tells it like it is. You can lose weight and regain your health and energy. You can wow the crowd, once you get honest with yourself about a few little habits.

Breathe a big sigh of relief. Each one of these habits is fixable. In the following pages, you'll learn which of your habits need a face-lift. You'll read stories from women just like you who have changed their lives by making a few simple tweaks in how they live. You'll hear about the research and learn what habits successful dieters—women who have lost weight and kept it off—adopt to stay trim and healthy for life. You'll also tailor a plan just right for you from hundreds of suggested simple steps, so that you can change your course from sabotage to success.

Embrace even a few of the simple steps in this book, change a habit or two, and you will reach your goals. You definitely will look and feel better. Hey, you might even fit back into your high school jeans or that little black dress!

Acknowledgments

To the hardcores who have seen me through many books—I thank my dear friend and agent, David Smith; my editor and bike buddy, Deborah Brody; and my research assistant, Victoria Dolby Toews. A special thanks to the friends, family members, clients, instructors, athletes, and students who so graciously offered their stories, advice, and confessions throughout this book. Most important of all, I thank my children, Lauren and Will, who patiently put up with their mother as she approached another deadline.

Without the expertise and research of some of this country's best nutrition experts and scientists and their willingness to answer my questions, I could not have written this book, nor any of my more than three hundred magazine articles and other books throughout the years. A sincere "thank you" to Dr. Edward Abramson at California State University at Chico; Dr. Tom Baranowski at Baylor College of Medicine; Dr. Lydia Bazzano at Beth Israel Deaconess Hospital; Dr. Jeffrey Blumberg at Tufts University; Dr. Dena M. Bravata at Stanford University School of Medicine; Dr. George Bray at Louisiana State University; Dr. Kelly Brownell at Yale University; Dr. Wayne C. Callaway at George Washington University; Dr. Larry Christensen at the University of South Alabama; Nancy Clark; Dr. Kenneth Cooper at the Cooper Institute of Aerobics Research; Dr. Winston Craig at Andrews University, in Michigan; Dr. Mary Dallman at the University of California, San Francisco; Mary Donkersloot; Dr. Adam Drewnowski at the University of Washington; Dr. Ken Druck; Dr. Robert H. Eckel at the University of Colorado Health Sciences Center; Sharon Edelstein at George Washington University; Anne Fletcher; Dr. John Foreyt at Baylor College of Medicine; Dr. Barry Goldin at Tufts University; Dr. Joseph Hibbeln at the National Institutes of Health; Gretchen Hill at Michigan State University; Dr. James Hill at the University of

Colorado Health Sciences Center; Dr. Bartley Hoebel at Princeton University; Dr. David Jenkins at the University of Toronto; Deborah Kesten; Dr. Susan Kleiner at the University of Washington; Dr. Richard Mattes at Purdue University; Kathy McManus at Brigham & Women's Hospital; Susan Moores; Carol Munter; Vince Nistico; Dr. Pamela Peeke at the University of Maryland School of Medicine; Dr. Suzanne Phelan at Brown University; Brenda Ponichtera; Judith Putnam at the USDA; Dr. Susan Roberts at Tufts University; Dr. Barbara Rolls at Pennsylvania State University; Dr. Paul Rozin at the University of Pennsylvania; Dr. Carmen D. Samuel-Hodge at the University of North Carolina; Dr. Howard D. Sesso at Harvard University; Dr. Jeffrey Sobal at Cornell University; Dr. Gary Stoner at Ohio State University; Dr. Amy Subar at the National Cancer Institute; Evelyn Tribole; Dr. Thomas Wadden at the University of Pennsylvania; Dr. Brian Wansink at the University of Illinois; Debra Waterhouse; Dr. Ronald Watson at the Arizona Health Sciences Center; Dr. Walter Willett at the Harvard School of Public Health; and Dr. Lisa Young at New York University.

Introduction:
The Scoop on Women's Diets

Reflect on your eating habits. How would you say you rate? Choose the description that best matches your diet:

___ **a.** Really good. I make healthful food choices almost all of the time.
___ **b.** Pretty good. I make healthful food choices most of the time.
___ **c.** Not so good. My unhealthy choices probably slightly outweigh the healthful ones.
___ **d.** Horrible. My food choices are a dietary train wreck. I love fast food, junk food, and chips; next to no healthful choices grace my lips.

If you're like most women, you probably rate your eating habits somewhere between "really good" and "pretty good." According to a Gallup poll conducted by Weight Watchers and the American Dietetic Association, 90 percent of women think their diets are reasonably healthy. Almost all of them are delusional.

The latest national nutrition survey of Americans' eating habits found that only one person out of every 100 of us meets even minimum standards of a balanced diet; the other 99 percent fall dismally short of optimal. According to a U.S. Department of Agriculture (USDA) study of women who rated their diets as excellent, less than 19 percent actually ate reasonably well.

If you want to be the healthiest you can be, if you want to finally lose the excess weight and fit into that little black dress again, if you really are serious about making changes for good, then it's time to get real and be honest, really honest, about what you're eating. Just in case you need a jolt of reality, here's a look at what the research has found most women put on their plates and into their bodies.

The Hourglass Diet

According to the latest data from the USDA, 70 percent of Americans say they are eating "pretty much whatever they want," up from 58 percent in the late 1990s. The foods that make up "whatever they want" are not the stuff of which healthy, trim bodies are made.

The Food Guide Pyramid, as shown in Figure I.1, outlines what a healthful diet should look like, with grains, fruits, and vegetables providing the greatest percentage of that diet, followed by moderate amounts of low-fat milk products and lean meats. That's not how most women eat. According to Judith Putnam, economist at the USDA Economic Research Service, in Washington, D.C., who tracks Americans' eating habits, we gobble lots of sugar and fat and platters of refined grains, but we sorely lack vegetables, fruits, low-fat milk products, and other nutritious foods. "It's no surprise that overall calories also are on the rise. We consume about 300 calories more every day than we did back in 1985," Putnam says. That's the equivalent of eating six extra chocolate chip cookies, 12 Hershey's Kisses, or an order of fries every day—a calorie excess that is sure to pack on the pounds.

We're Eating Too Much

It's no secret why we gain weight. "We're eating more calories and moving less than we did even 20 years ago," says John Foreyt, Ph.D., director of the Nutrition Research Center at Baylor College of Medicine, in Houston. Part of the problem is the food we choose. Compared with our parents' generation, we consume lots more sugar, refined grains, and processed or fast foods.

- **Sugar:** We currently average 158 pounds of sugar per woman per year. No one has ever eaten this much sugar before in the

Figure I.1

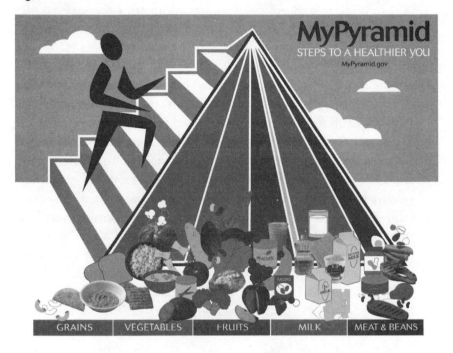

history of the planet. If you're like many women, you up the ante when you're feeling gloomy or depressed, and during the 10 days to two weeks before your period, gobbling an additional 20 percent of calories from fat and sugar!

- **Grains:** Our muffins and scones are the size of small cakes, and our bagels are closer to five portions of grain than they are to one portion. Pasta is served on platters, not plates, in restaurants. So, it's no wonder the latest USDA figures show we are averaging closer to 11 servings a day of grains, most of them highly refined and nutrient-defunct.
- **Fat:** For several years, we cut back a bit on fat. That trend is over. As women jump on the latest low-carb diet fad, fat consumption is back on the rise, increasing our risk for heart disease, cancer, and other ills.
- **Fast food:** Two out of every five of us regularly eat fast food. These foods, along with store-bought processed foods, are

packed with sugar and fat and are less filling. They also are often supersized, so we eat more, adding unnecessary calories before we feel satisfied.

Study after study has found that the more processed and refined foods women eat, the more likely we are to consume poor diets and to gain weight. A study from the Harvard School of Public Health found that on days when people eat fast food, they consume an average of 187 excess calories (equates to a 6-pound weight gain during one year), and eating fast food more than twice a week is enough to increase a woman's risk of being over-weight by 86 percent. On days when we eat typical fast-food fare—hamburgers, fries, chicken nuggets, meat and cheese burritos, colas, milkshakes, and so on—our intake of added sugar, fat, salt, and calories is higher (see Figure I.2), while our intake of fiber, calcium-rich milk, fruits, and vegetables drops.

Another study, from the USDA Research Service, in Beltsville, Maryland, found the same thing—people who eat fast food consume diets too high in calories and are most likely to be over-weight. Typical fast-food fare is so greasy that one meal alone adds a third of a woman's daily requirements for calories, fat, and saturated fat. You don't have to be a junk-food junkie; even once-a-week trips to the drive-through add up. In short, calories increase and nutrients decrease with every single fast-food meal.

We're Not Eating Enough

It's not just *what* we are eating that is getting us into trouble; it's also what we're *not* eating, such as sufficient amounts of fruits and vegetables (as well as nuts, beans, whole grains, nonfat milk, and other real foods), the very foods that keep us well, help us look younger and feel our best, and ensure that we keep our girlish figures.

With the deck stacked so high in favor of eating the likes of chin-dribbling strawberries and mouth-watering watermelon, you'd think we'd be shoveling handfuls of orange slices into our mouths, blending gallons of strawberries into smoothies, and

Figure I.2

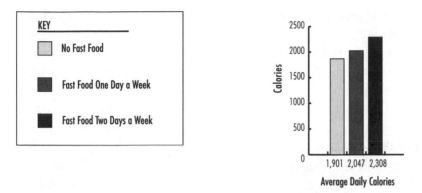

KEY

☐ No Fast Food

■ Fast Food One Day a Week

■ Fast Food Two Days a Week

Average Daily Calories

1,901 2,047 2,308

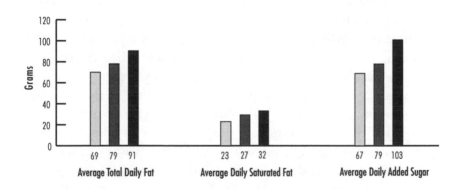

Average Total Daily Fat

69 79 91

Average Daily Saturated Fat

23 27 32

Average Daily Added Sugar

67 79 103

fighting over the last asparagus spear at the dinner table. We're not. In fact, it's just the opposite. Most women think they eat enough produce, but they actually average only about four servings a day of fruits and vegetables, and more than half of all women don't eat fruit at all on any given day. Our average daily consumption has inched up only 0.3 serving since the 1970s, the equivalent of an extra bite of a banana. Fruits and vegetables account for only 8 percent of that 300-calories-a-day increase mentioned earlier. The rest comes from ballooning portions of meat and from refined and sweetened grains. Few women over the age of 18 can lose weight on that kind of diet! Even fewer can rest assured that they are healthy.

We do no better when it comes to whole grains. While we eat record amounts of refined grains, typical consumption of whole grains is less than one serving a day. Eighty-five percent of our grains are refined, which contributes to a huge fiber shortfall, not to mention the vitamins and minerals that are lost when grains are processed. "Whole grains also supply health-enhancing phytochemicals not found in refined grains," adds Jeffrey Blumberg, Ph.D., professor in the Friedman School of Nutrition Science and Policy at Tufts University, in Boston. Many refined grains, such as cakes, cookies, doughnuts, and muffins, are so high in fat that they rank number four as a source of saturated fat in our diets. Research repeatedly reports that women who eat the most whole grains have lower risks for stroke, colon cancer, diabetes, high blood pressure, and heart disease. They also are more likely to maintain a healthy weight, and if they gain weight, they have an easier time losing it, compared with women who turn to white bread, white rice, and other refined grains for their carbs.

Beans also are on our black list, yet they are so good for us. Beans make it to the plate more often today than in the early '90s, but women still average only about a cup a year, a pittance compared with the 50 pounds of pork we gobble at the same time. Beans and other legumes (split peas, lentils) are cholesterol-free, almost fat-free, and rich in fiber and nutrients, supplying more than half a day's requirement for folic acid and hefty amounts of calcium, magnesium, iron, and zinc in every serving. They also are loaded with phytochemicals, such as saponins and phytosterols, that lower cancer and heart disease risk, and they are low in the glycemic index, so they help regulate blood sugar, as well as appetite. "Increasing bean intake as part of a diet rich in fruits and vegetables might help prevent heart disease, lower cholesterol, and even lower blood pressure," says Lydia Bazzano, M.D., Ph.D., Harvard Clinical Fellow in Medicine at Beth Israel Deaconess Hospital. Bazzano's study found that people who included beans in their diets at least four times a week lowered their heart-disease risk by 22 percent, compared with people whose diets included a serving or less each week.

Nuts are high in calories, so they often are the first to go when a woman goes on a weight-loss diet, yet nuts of all kinds are too good for us to ignore. An ounce of nuts added to the diet several times a week could cut your risk for heart disease by up to 39 percent, as well as lower cancer and diabetes risk. If you're like most Americans, you're averaging less than an ounce of nuts a week, so you are depriving yourself of a rich source of protein, magnesium, vitamin E, potassium, fiber, and B vitamins. Granted, nuts are high in calories, but the fat in most nuts is heart-healthy monounsaturated fat and appears to help with weight loss. "When people include moderate amounts of favorite fatty foods in their diets, such as peanut butter or canola oil in stir-fries, they enjoy food more and don't feel that they are dieting, even though they are losing weight," says Kathy McManus, M.S., R.D., at Brigham & Women's Hospital, in Boston.

It seems that the more nutritious a food is, the less we want to eat it. Take wheat germ, for example. Anyone under 55 typically shuns this little nutrition nugget, with consumption on the decline since 2002. Yet, the heart of the wheat kernel is a gold mine of nutrients. A half-cup serving of toasted wheat germ supplies more than half of your daily magnesium needs, as well as husky amounts of vitamins, including 100 percent of your daily need for folic acid and 50 percent of your vitamin E requirement. Wheat germ also supplies decent amounts of trace minerals, such as iron and zinc.

It's true that we are making an effort when it comes to some healthy foods, such as soy milk and yogurt. Soy milk has moved from the fringes to mainstream, yet regular consumption increased only 3 percent in 2003, according to the Soyfoods Association of North America, and only one in every six women consumes a glass or more a week. This simple way to add soy to the diet packs a major nutrient punch. Fortified soy milk is a great alternative to cow's milk in supplying calcium and vitamin D, and it contains phytoestrogens that lower heart disease risk, possibly reduces the risk for memory loss and osteoporosis, and even might help with weight loss.

Yogurt consumption is on the rise, too, but daily intake still hovers at only about 2 tablespoons. "Low-fat yogurt is a healthy food, supplying protein, B vitamins, and calcium. It's a useful alternative to milk for people who are lactose intolerant, and if it contains the probiotic bacteria, such as *Lactobacillus acidophilus* or *bifidobacterium*, it helps prevent GI-tract problems like constipation and diarrhea, as well as helping to treat food allergies," says Barry Goldin, Ph.D., in the Department of Family Medicine and Community Health at Tufts. These healthful bacteria wade past the stomach and flourish in the intestinal tract, according to Goldin. They crowd out disease-causing bacteria, produce natural antibiotics, and possibly switch off an enzyme that triggers colon cancer.

We've also cut back on our meat and whole-milk intake, probably because we are more aware that these foods are high in saturated fat and increase our risk for heart disease and cancer. However, we've more than made up the difference by gobbling three times as much cheese, which, ounce-for-ounce, is much higher in saturated fat than either meat or milk. "It's interesting that whenever people lower their fat intake in one area, the fat just pops up someplace else," says Judith Putnam. Cheese now outranks meat as the number one source of saturated fat in the diet. Two-thirds of that cheese is added to our fast foods and processed foods, from burritos, tacos, nachos, and cheeseburgers to salads, pizza, sauces for baked potatoes, packaged snack foods, and fries.

Get a Real Food Life: The Six Preplanning Steps to Eating Well

The good news is that when you eat well, when you feast on fruits, vegetables, whole grains, legumes, and other real foods, and when you fix the little habits that subtly undermine your best efforts to eat healthy, you automatically lose weight without even trying. You reclaim your health as you fit back into those too-tight jeans. It's also a relief to know that it takes only a few minor changes in what you're eating to produce big-time results. For example, Dr. Amy Subar, Ph.D., R.D., research nutritionist at the National Cancer Institute in Bethesda, Maryland, says, "If women focused on increasing their vegetables and fruits and minimizing added fats such as butter, margarine, and cream, especially when eating out, they would be well on their way to eating better."

Getting a grip on your eating habits and raising your diet score from a "pretty good" to a "really good," or even from "horrible" to "pretty good," begins with six basic preplanning steps. Keep in mind that changing your eating habits is more about attitude and commitment than it is about grocery lists, vitamins, or calorie counting. If you want to feel your best—energized, gorgeous, vital, and leaner—you must believe you can do it and make the process a priority.

Step 1: Do It for You

The deciding moment for many women who got serious about eating well was when they realized that the process of making healthful food choices or losing weight was up to them. These women failed at past attempts because they weren't making the changes for themselves, but rather were doing it for a spouse, a sister's wedding, or a class reunion. "Once they realized that there was no magic bullet and that the buck stopped here, they accepted that their desire to be healthier or to manage their weight was a lifelong process within their power," says Anne Fletcher, M.S., R.D., author of *Thin for Life*. They decided that the changes they must make for life were worth it for themselves, their health, their well-being, and their self-respect. As a result, they dropped the "why me" mantra. "It isn't fair that some people have to be more careful with their diets, to move more or eat less than others, but that's the reality," says Jim Hill, Ph.D., professor of pediatrics and medicine at the University of Colorado Health Sciences Center. He adds, "The sooner a woman accepts that and gets to the real question of what to do about it, the better."

Take a long, hard look at whom you are making the dietary changes for. Only when you honestly can say that you are doing it "for me" are you ready to begin a healthier eating plan or to lose weight and keep it off. You also must accept the fact that there are no magic pills, diet gurus, food combinations, or products, gizmos, or gadgets that can do it for you. "You can't kid yourself about your weight, how much you eat or exercise, or how you look. You must own the problem and get honest with yourself about what you're doing and what you'll need to do to change," says Fletcher.

Step 2: Get Ready for a Whole New You

It takes courage to break old patterns, connect with different people, and develop new pastimes. Revamp your life, and you open new horizons, while closing a few old (dysfunctional) doors. Hill says, "Anyone who has lost 60 or more pounds and kept it off, or made significant changes in what she eats and how much she exercises, is a different person, with a new life, new friends, and new ways to spend free time." You still have the tried-and-true old buddies, but you now visit with them at home over a cup of tea instead of at a restaurant over a full meal. You've also made new friends on your Wednesday-night bike rides. "My family adjusted over time to a meat-and-three-vegetables dinner, which was a big accomplishment considering we used to eat fast food four times a week," says Robin, the mother of grown children and a teacher in Reno. Family time is now time spent throwing Frisbees or shooting hoops instead of watching TV; the lunch hour is spent with a different set of coworkers, who walk instead of eat; and you get excited about a tasty way to cook eggplant, rather than another calorie-packed cheesecake recipe.

Make it as easy as possible on yourself by linking the new "healthy you" with something that's already important in your life. "For some, their food preparation time is their spiritual time, or they hook exercise with socializing," says Hill. To motivate yourself, use nonfood rewards for daily accomplishments, such as stars on a calendar, new clothes, a movie, or an hour to read a good book. Remember the "if . . . then" rule: If you accomplish a goal (e.g., replace the butter on your toast with all-fruit jam, skip dessert, or add one extra serving of vegetables), then—and only then—do you get the reward.

Step 3: Practice, Not Perfect

"Women who successfully maintain a healthy eating style are vigilant in their efforts. They essentially nip any slips in healthful eating or weight regain in the bud, day by day and meal by meal," says Foreyt. Although the method varies, healthy eaters know that setbacks are inevitable, and they have attack plans in place to quickly handle slips. They keep records of their food intake, return to their healthy-eating efforts at the first sign of a 1- to 5-pound weight gain, and/or count calories or fat grams. Some quit baking or cut out desserts; others watch portions or schedule exercise sessions as if they were appointments. "The good news is that healthy eaters consistently report that it gets easier over time. It's a practice-makes-perfect scenario, so if you maintain the new habits for more than two years, you're likely to stick with it for life," says Suzanne Phelan, Ph.D., coinvestigator in the National Weight Control Registry (NWCR) and assistant professor of psychology at Brown University.

Be aware of small slips in your healthy-eating efforts or gains in weight, and have a specific plan that will immediately get you back on track. Perhaps you notice that your dessert servings are increasing or that you're nibbling more and more from your partner's bag of french fries. Maybe you realize that the lettuce is wilting in the refrigerator rather than making it to your plate, that you're finding more excuses not to eat well, or that your goal to eat three fruits every day has dwindled to a reality of just two servings. The plan to get back on track will vary from person to person but could include journal keeping, weighing and measuring your food, a halt on alcoholic beverages, focusing more on fruits and vegetables, setting new goals, deciding to eat only the food you have portioned onto your own plate, or not entering the kitchen after supper until you're back to eating well again.

Step 4: Handle Emotions Without Food

Stress is a main cause of relapse and poor eating. Numerous studies, including ones from the University of Oxford and Fairfield University, in Connecticut, found that people who stick with healthy eating habits believe themselves capable of handling problems and are direct in solving difficulties, compared with unsuccessful dieters who avoid or escape adversity and turn to food for solace. Women who stick with a healthy eating plan know that it's about talking to yourself in a supportive, encouraging way. It's about asking for what you need. It's about getting in touch with feelings. "Women who in the past typically put others' needs in front of their own, stuffed [suppressed] stress, and then rewarded themselves with food at the end of the day find that if they get in touch with how they are feeling, are a little more selfish about allowing time to exercise and to eat right, and are more assertive in asking for what they want are much more likely to stick with a healthy eating plan or to keep the weight off," says Fletcher.

The critical first step is to identify and label your emotions. "Ask yourself if it's fatigue, anger, anxiety, a need for comfort, or true hunger that is triggering a desire to eat the wrong foods. Food will solve only a hunger problem; in all other cases, the solution lies elsewhere," says Fletcher. The next step is to develop self-empowering skills, such as assertive communication, positive self-talk, and ways to relax, to constructively nip stress in the bud. Instead of snuggling up with a gallon of ice cream, learn how to explain to people the way you feel, go for a walk to let off steam, get together with a friend, or forget the chores and go to a movie when times get rough.

Step 5: Measure Success

Success isn't about eating perfectly or reaching your ideal weight; it's about reaching a balance in your life. Most healthy eaters still nibble on chips or cookies or are slightly heavier than they set out to be. "If you saw them on the street, you wouldn't say they were thin," says Fletcher. Perfection is too hard to maintain. Instead, set a realistic goal so you're not hungry all the time, obsessed with foods you can't have, or so consumed with exercise that you don't have a life. Even small changes over time can have big payoffs. "Women who eat well, but not perfectly, still report tremendous improvements in their quality of life despite not achieving their ultimate goal," says Phelan. They are leaner, fitter, happier, and more confident than in days past, and they keep at it without falling back to unhealthy eating habits.

Too often, women make unrealistic goals that set them up for failure. A comfortable body weight or a healthy diet is one you can maintain without obsessing over food 24-7, yet you still feel good. Create a clear picture in your mind of what you ultimately want your diet to look like, how you want to feel and look as a result of eating that way, and how your life in general will be different. Perhaps you see yourself with more energy, enthusiasm for life, and vitality. You might visualize yourself looking healthier, with clearer, more youthful skin. Your goal might be to enjoy socializing with friends or family over healthy fare. Images of fueling your body with foods on which it thrives or of a leaner, more fit body shape might represent one of your goals. Then divide that goal into little, manageable steps, such as including three servings of whole grains in your daily menu, limiting your fast food or soft drinks to twice a week, or refraining from eating off others' plates. Plan to take one or more years to make all the changes and to reach your vision.

Step 6: Live It Up

Eating well is not about deprivation or denial. In fact, women who have mastered the art of eating well and losing weight say they've never felt so good and so in control and satisfied with their lives. They enjoy food, socializing, and cooking. They enjoy how their new bodies look and feel. They give themselves permission to be imperfect, and they treat themselves—but only on occasion, not constantly, and with smaller portions. They satisfy their cravings with a cookie or a few chips, not the entire bag, and they control high-risk items, such as cheese and chocolate, by not keeping them in the house. Their taste buds have changed with time, so that they crave mangos or strawberries and are sickened by greasy foods. It's also about trade-offs. "You might choose to have a slice of pizza or a glass of wine, but then forgo dessert," says Fletcher. These diet successes have developed skills for creating full lives, ones that bring joy and meet their needs, so they don't turn to food for solace. "Women who have incorporated healthful eating habits into their lives have changed for good, and when they make that switch, success happens. They feel good, have more energy, are proud of themselves, and are more self-assured, and so it's no surprise that they enjoy life more," says Foreyt.

Make conscious decisions about how to spend your daily calorie allotment. If dark chocolate is your favorite treat, then have a small piece, but don't waste your time on a less-satisfying bologna sandwich. Take time out of a busy day to nurture yourself in nonfood ways, such as having a pedicure or a hot bath. Most important, put the food-and-diet thing into perspective. When you reach the end of your days and take stock of your life, heaven forbid that your main accomplishment was that you agonized over your diet!

What Does Healthy Eating Look Like?

You need a goal to work toward, and that means having a clear image in your head of what should be on your plate most of the time. Throw out the fad nutrition books that propose bizarre eating habits, such as food combining, or that blame a food group, such as carbs, for all your problems, from diabetes and fatigue to weight gain and wrinkling. Instead, stick to what thousands of studies spanning decades of research have proven over and over to be the only way to eat well, stay optimally healthy, and keep your girlish figure.

Most women who have found that balance between eating well and living realistically have learned to monitor calories and portions, eat lots of produce and quality carbs, and limit fat grams. "They also eat consistently, regardless of whether it's a weekday, weekend, or holiday," says Phelan. They eat at least three meals a day, and many include a few snacks, too. "Ask these women what is different about their diets today compared with the past, and they overwhelmingly respond that they used to eat haphazardly and now make a concerted effort to eat regular meals," says Fletcher. For example, 8 out of every 10 women in the NWCR, an ongoing research study of people who have lost weight and maintained the weight loss, report eating breakfast every day.

The eating plan is simple: The mainstays of a healthy woman's diet are vegetables and fruit; breads, cereals, and pasta (mostly whole grain); and legumes. Along with that, include moderate amounts of nonfat or low-fat milk products or soy milk, chicken breast, nuts, and fish, and small amounts, if any, of extra-lean meats. Most women who have successfully conquered the diet struggle also limit or cut out fast-food restaurants. Nine out of 10 eat low-fat fare, watch portions, eat regular meals beginning with breakfast, and listen to their bodies, eating when hungry and stopping when comfortably full.

It's the putting into practice of these guidelines that varies. "When I asked women what their three most important diet habits were, I got 90 different answers—a testament to the importance of tailoring an eating plan to your personal likes and lifestyle," says Fletcher. In short, don't define how you eat as *dieting*, but rather as a consistent eating plan that you live with for life.

The Ultimate Diet Plan

Every day, aim for the following foods and servings. These guidelines ensure that you consume 100 percent of all the vitamins, minerals, fiber, protein, healthy fats, and phytochemicals you need to feel, look, and be your best today and for the rest of your life. It may seem like a lot of food, but real foods are nutrient-packed, not caloric-dense. You'll be getting only about 1,500 to 1,800 calories a day on the following foods. If you are active and can have more calories, add more servings of these foods or a few treats to the menu.

Vegetables and Fruits

(*Goal*: eight or more servings a day)
Most women need to double or even triple their current intake of fruits and vegetables to meet minimum standards. To start,

include two fruits or vegetables at every meal and one at every snack. Select mostly deep-colored produce, such as carrots, sweet potatoes, spinach, blueberries, dried plums, and green peas. Choose only 100 percent juice, such as orange, grapefruit, or pineapple juice. Mix and match raw vegetables and fruits for salads and snacks with cooked produce and dried fruit.

Grains

(*Goal*: a minimum of six servings daily; at least three should be whole grains)

According to the USDA's Healthy Eating Index—which ranks Americans' eating habits from 1 to 10 in 10 categories, for a perfect score of 100—we earn a grade of D for grains, averaging only 6 out of 10 points. Focus on whole grains. Choose whole-wheat bread, brown rice, and plain oatmeal instead of white bread, white rice, and granola bars. Skip the contents of the pastry case in favor of air-popped popcorn, baked corn chips, and whole-wheat crackers. Sprinkle wheat germ into batters for pancakes, waffles, muffins, and breads. Use whole-wheat flour when possible.

Nonfat Milk or Fortified Soy Milk

(*Goal*: three servings a day, 1,000 to 1,200 mg of calcium)

Only one out of every five women consumes enough calcium from milk, with most women averaging about one and a half servings a day and a little more than 600 mg of calcium. Include at least three fat-free or low-fat, calcium-rich foods in the daily menu, such as nonfat or 1 percent low-fat milk or yogurt, fortified soy milk or orange juice, and canned salmon. Otherwise, take a 500 mg calcium supplement to fill in the gaps.

Legumes, Fish, Poultry Breast

(*Goal*: two to three servings a day)

Beans are gold mines of vitamins, trace minerals, fiber, and heart-healthy phytochemicals. They also help manage your weight because they fill you up before they fill you out. Limit red

What Should My Diet Look Like?

The Basics—Every Day, You Should Eat:
   8+ fruits and vegetables
   6 grains (3 whole grain)
   3 calcium-rich foods
   2 legumes, meat, chicken, fish

Breakfast: 1 whole grain, 1 calcium-rich food, 2 fruits or vegetables
   Such as:
      1 cup of whole-wheat cereal topped with ¼ cup of dried cranberries
      1 cup of nonfat milk or calcium-fortified soy milk
      1 small banana

Lunch: 2 grains, 1 meat or legume, 1 calcium-rich food, 2 fruits or vegetables
   Such as:
      Turkey sandwich on whole-wheat bread
      2 cups of tossed salad with low-fat dressing
      1 glass of nonfat milk or calcium-fortified soy milk

Dinner: 2 grains, 1 meat or legume, 2 fruits or vegetables
   Such as:
      1 3-ounce serving of fish, chicken breast, or lean meat
      1 sweet potato
      ½ cup of green peas
      ½ cup of wild rice

Snacks: 2 fruits or vegetables, 1 grain, 1 calcium-rich food
   Such as:
      Banana
      Orange
      Graham crackers
      Fruited low-fat yogurt

meat, and add one to two servings of beans per week, such as kidney beans in salads, fat-free refried beans in burritos, and hummus spread for sandwiches. Include two fish dishes in the weekly plan, such as baked salmon, tuna salad, or grilled-fish tacos to supply heart-healthy omega-3 fats.

Oils and Fats

(*Limit intake.*)
We've cut back a little on butter and margarine, but we are eating record amounts of vegetable oils. In fact, salad dressing is the number one source of fat in women's diets. "What is startling is that our intake of added fats [margarine, salad oils, butter, fats used to process foods, etc.] totals almost all the fat a woman should consume in order to fall within the limits of a 30 percent fat diet," says Putnam. Add to that the fats in meat and dairy, and . . . oops, we've blown our low-fat diets. Besides the unnecessary calories, the more fat a woman eats, the less likely she is to get enough vegetables, fruit, whole grains, fish, nonfat milk, vitamins C and A, folic acid, and fiber. So, choose unprocessed foods, such as baked potatoes, instead of french fries or chips; whole-wheat bread instead of a scone or croissant; and grilled instead of fried foods. Use low-fat or fat-free salad dressing and mayonnaise, and moderate amounts of olive oil, and limit cookies, pastries, processed snack items, and most fast foods to once a week, since these sweet treats often contain more fat than sugar. One exception to this rule is nuts; you can include up to an ounce a day to lower disease risk and help manage weight. Read labels and select only those processed foods that contain no more than 3 grams of fat per 100 calories.

Added Sugar

(*Goal*: Limit added sugars to about 7 percent of calories—6 teaspoons for a 1,600-calorie diet, 12 teaspoons for a 2,200-calorie diet.)

Sugar intake has never been so high. Much of our sugar comes from the 54 gallons of soft drinks—the number one source of sugar—that we each drink annually. The other three-quarters of our sugar is hidden in processed foods, from fruited yogurts to flavored oatmeal. Instead, limit soda to one or two 12-ounce cans a week. Limit pastries and desserts. Read labels: avoid foods that list sugar as one of the first three ingredients or that contain several types of sugar, such as sucrose, high-fructose corn syrup, and glucose. (Hint: There are 4 grams in every teaspoon of sugar, so a product that lists sugar content as 26 grams contains 6½ teaspoons of sugar.)

Those 10 Habits

If I told you I had a pill that would slow aging; help prevent every age-related disease from heart disease, diabetes, hypertension, and cancer to memory loss, frailty, and feebleness; help you feel and look younger for the rest of your life; have no side effects other than improved mood, energy level, and self-image; and be the secret to a leaner figure and a more youthful appearance, would you take it? You'd be crazy not to! Well, it may not be a pill, but a few simple changes in your diet (and exercise) will provide all those benefits and more.

So, what's stopping you from shedding your old ways and blossoming into the healthy woman you are supposed to be? My guess is there is a habit or two, maybe one of which you're not even aware of, that subtly undermines your best intentions to eat well or stay fit. That little habit is probably a bit unconscious, although if I were to catch you doing it, you'd say, "Oh, I know I shouldn't do that, but I don't do it very often; a little won't hurt." Maybe the habit is saying no to having a piece of the apricot coffee cake on the kitchen counter but later taking a bite every time you walk by. Maybe it's having that one cola every afternoon for a pick-me-up. Maybe it's finishing off the french fries on your kids' plates at restaurants.

The good news is that habits are learned, so they can be unlearned or replaced with new habits that support your desire to fulfill your vision of being energized, vital, sexy, healthy, and lean. The first step in this self-discovery is recognizing what that little habit is doing to your efforts. The next few chapters will blow the whistle on our most common dietary stumbling blocks and, most important, explain what to do about them.

How Does Your Diet Rate, Habitwise?

Be honest. Do you sometimes skip breakfast? Order a burger and fries from the drive-through? Grab a bag of chips and a soft drink for a snack? Have you tried more than four fad diets in the past 10 years? Given up carbs, only to sneak a bag of cookies when no one is looking? Do you eat off others' plates, from the fridge, and out of the pan? Now is the time to really take a look at the habits that might jeopardize your health and waistline. No need to show this assessment to anyone. Answer the questions (honestly!), and then score your points to see how you rate and what habits might be doing you in. Rank your answers 0 to 2:

    0 = Never
    1 = Sometimes
    2 = Always

__ 1. I serve myself reasonable portions and never eat leftovers on others' plates, nibble while cleaning the kitchen or cooking, or snack from the pan, from the refrigerator, or out of the serving bowl.

__ 2. I make food choices based on what I know is best for me; when I am eating with friends or family, I always include at least two foods that I consider healthy and good for me.

___ 3. At restaurants, I order low-fat, healthy foods and watch portions.

___ 4. I am honest about what and how much I eat, and I know the approximate portion sizes and calories for my favorite foods.

___ 5. I include at least eight servings of fruits and/or vegetables, not counting french fries or other fried potatoes, in my daily menu.

___ 6. I choose only dark-colored produce, such as romaine lettuce, spinach, blueberries, carrots, orange juice, cantaloupe, sweet potatoes, and broccoli.

___ 7. I eat consciously and have a specific plan for how and what I want to eat and how much I want to exercise every day.

___ 8. I recognize that my food choices, body weight, and fitness level are my choices and my responsibility and that I can't blame my hormones, glands, the time clock, or anyone else for these choices.

___ 9. I eat when I'm physically hungry, not because I'm bored, tired, anxious, or stressed or for any emotional reason.

___ 10. I have coping skills to handle adversity, so I don't turn to food for solace.

___ 11. I eat at least three whole grains a day, including whole-grain breads, cereals, pastas, and crackers.

___ 12. I average three servings daily of nonfat milk, milk products, and/or calcium-fortified soy milk, cheese, or orange juice.

___ 13. I average two to three protein-rich foods every day, and my choices are poultry breast, fish, and/or legumes.

___ 14. I limit fats; what fats I do eat come from nuts, seeds, olive or canola oil, avocados, fish, olives, and/or nut butters.

continued

___ 15. I use fat-free or low-fat salad dressings and mayonnaise.

___ 16. I avoid processed foods that contain added fats, such as fried foods, snack items, and convenience or fast foods.

___ 17. I select only foods with little or no added sugars.

___ 18. I eat minimeals and snacks throughout the day, so that no more than four hours will go by between meals.

___ 19. I eat a breakfast that includes a grain, a fruit, and a calcium- or protein-rich food, such as eggs, milk, or peanut butter.

___ 20. I bake, steam, broil, poach, or grill food, rather than fry, sauté, or use sauces and gravies that contain added fat.

___ 21. I avoid fad diets; when I need to drop a few pounds, I return to sensible eating habits—real food, not processed foods—and increase my exercise.

___ 22. I take a moderate-dose multiple vitamin and mineral supplement.

___ 23. I drink alcohol in moderation or not at all (no more than one drink a day).

___ 24. I drink at least eight glasses of water every day.

___ 25. I give myself credit for small accomplishments and don't ruin my healthy-eating efforts by falling off the wagon at the first slip or weight gain.

Score:

37 to 50: Outstanding. You have conquered many of the habits that typically interfere with women's health, diets, and weight-loss efforts. You can stick with your current eating plan, or aim for turning one or two lower scores into a "2."

25 to 36: Average. You have fallen into some bad habits that are roadblocks to feeling and looking your best. Identify three or four "0" and "1" scores that you want to boost into the next higher range. When you've successfully accomplished this, tackle two or three more.

0 to 24: Oops. Time to start taking your health more seriously. Set a goal to gradually improve your score by 3 points every month.

If you scored lower than 2 on this question:	*Make sure you thoroughly read this chapter:*
1	1
2, 3	2
4	3
5, 6	4
7	5
8	6
9, 10	7
11–22	8
23, 24	9
25	10

Mindless Eating

"I don't eat anything; I don't understand why I can't lose weight." Laura was obviously frustrated and discouraged as she voiced these words. She'd answered all my questions correctly: She didn't use much fat in her diet. She ate lots of fruits and vegetables. She watched her portions. She had cut back on sugar and processed foods. She seldom, if ever, ventured into a fast-food restaurant.

Something wasn't right. No one defies the laws of physics by gaining weight on veggies and grilled chicken. So, I followed Laura for a day. I wrote down everything she put into her mouth, and then I tallied the results. Sure enough, everything she had told me was true. It was what she *hadn't* fessed up to that was causing the weight gain.

Laura cleaned up the kitchen after her three boys had eaten breakfast. She finished off the leftover toast and the bits of scrambled egg, and drank the last few gulps of milk before putting the glasses in the dishwasher. "I hate to see food go to waste," she explained. She then ate the nutritious breakfast she had described to me, one that included a bowl of cereal and fruit. At work, she grabbed a cup of coffee with cream, finished off a bite of doughnut left in the employees' lounge, and ate a chocolate kiss as she passed by a worker's desk (she ate three more during the rest of the day), in addition to having her turkey sandwich, tossed salad, and yogurt at lunch. When she arrived home that evening, she nibbled on the last bit of a PB&J sandwich and pieces of a sugar cookie remaining in the kids' lunch boxes as she began preparing dinner. Laura tasted the sauce as she cooked, poured the milk for dinner and then finished off what wouldn't fit in the glasses by drinking it straight from the carton, and ate the end of the bread as she sliced a loaf for dinner. All told, that day Laura consumed a reasonable 1,800 calories in food served on a plate, and an additional 700 calories in foods randomly and unconsciously nibbled, grazed, and grabbed one bite at a time. No wonder she couldn't understand why she was gaining weight . . . almost 40 percent of her daily calorie intake was consumed unconsciously! Most of those unconscious calories came from sugar and fat.

Women's relationships with food can be divided into two categories: the foods chosen when our minds are engaged, and the foods nibbled and noshed mindlessly. When it comes to the former category, like Laura, most of us try to make good choices, and as discussed in the Introduction, up to 90 percent of us truly think we're doing a pretty good job. The latter category contains food that are almost always high in fat, sugar, and calories and low in the nutrients on which our bodies thrive. "If we had hidden cameras that followed us around all day, we would be shocked at the level of mindless eating we do," says Debra Waterhouse, M.P.H., R.D., author of *Outsmarting the Mother-Daughter Food Trap*. If you can't lose weight no matter how hard you try, or you're not as healthy as you would like, this mindless eating is the first place to check.

Invisible Calories

"Women are masters at mindless eating both inside and outside the home," says Susan Moores, M.S., R.D., spokesperson for the American Dietetic Association. We nibble off of a partner's plate, taste-test while cooking, and take a fork to an entire cake without cutting a piece. Taste-testing at the grocery store is a great way to pack away a few hundred calories. My daughter, Lauren, loves to go to Costco, not to shop, but to fill up on the taste-treat samples.

In some unconscious way, we consider this to be "free" food in every sense. It wasn't served in a dish, portioned into a bowl, or eaten at the table, and the nibbling wasn't even watched by anyone taller than three feet, so it doesn't count. "I am most likely to overeat after dinner when there are leftovers but not really enough to keep. I hate to throw food away, so I eat it instead. I've heard the saying 'Better to waste than to waist,' but it hasn't sunk in," says Angela, the mother of three small children in Woodside, California.

Here are a few primary, but certainly not all-encompassing, places where we are likely to nosh:

- **In the kitchen.** We are usually the primary chefs at home, which places us in a handy position to eat. It's no wonder that women pack in the calories just preparing and cleaning up in the minutes surrounding meals. We grab an extra handful of cheese to pop into our mouths as we sprinkle the rest over the lasagna, and we all but lick the plates as we clean up. We also eat spoonfuls of cookie dough, pie filling, and cake or pudding scrapings. What we forget to consider is that every spoonful of cookie dough packs a 70-calorie wallop, which, if eaten every day, equates to a 7-pound weight gain in one year. A potato chip, a french fry, a spoonful of spaghetti sauce, a taste-test of mashed potatoes—any of these nibbles may pack only about 10 to 20 calories. But, who has just one chip and just one taste? Repeatedly tasting, nibbling, and munching adds up. In the same way, just cutting out this mindless eating could be the very ticket to health.
- **When dining out.** Restaurants are another haven for mindless eating. "You seldom see men eating off of each other's plates at a restaurant, but the food on any man's plate that's within 50 feet of a woman is fair game," says Moores. Sometimes those nibbles are in addition to what's already on our own plates; other times we don't even bother to order an entree, having the full intent from the moment we sit down to graze off others' meals. "At restaurants, I have my entree, which is

usually a salad or grilled salmon, but I always reach across the table to take french fries or a sparerib off my husband's plate," says Dolores, a retired government worker in Oregon, who adds that she is the worst when it comes to sweets. "I won't order dessert, because I'm watching calories, but I ask my husband to order the chocolate cheesecake so I can have a bite. More often than not, I have a lot more than a taste."

- **With the kids.** When caring for children, we take mindless nibbling to an all-time high. Even women who wouldn't dream of nibbling anywhere else are likely to pop this or that into their mouths when they are caring for children. "Since having kids, I find myself constantly nibbling," says Elizabeth, the mother of two young girls in Dallas. We finish off the last of the kids' sandwiches, eat the last third of a child's piece of birthday cake, bite-by-bite finish off their pizza crust, nibble on the ravioli while serving dinner, and dole out the snack in a one-for-you-and-one-for-me style. Most kids are still in tune with their satiety signals and know when they are full, so they leave food on the plate, which is then ripe for the taking. Maybe the problem is that we are focused on feeding and providing snacks to our kids, so the opportunity to eat is more frequent. Maybe it's that kid-friendly foods, such as grilled cheese sandwiches, are not our typical fare, so they are exceptionally tempting. Besides, we have served our children healthy food, so even if it ends up in our bodies, we can gloat over what a fine job we are doing as nurturing parents! "I completely ignore the fact that I am taking two bites of mac and cheese, a graham cracker, a cheese goldfish cracker, or a spoonful of yogurt. If we go to a party with the kids, and I am helping serve one of them, I mindlessly put a few chips on my kid's plate and stick a few in my mouth before ever contemplating what I am going to have," Elizabeth adds. One woman said she was ready to buy a dog after her kids were born so that someone else in the house could take over the job of garbage disposal.

- **At the movies.** Combine an engrossing movie, the comfort of the dark, and tasty food, and you have the perfect opportunity for mindless eating. Anyone is likely to overeat at the movies given half a chance, but women take the cake. In some cases, the catalyst seems to be the container. "Women eat 40 percent more if served popcorn in a supersized bucket than if given a large bag. We even gave them stale popcorn, and they ate 45 percent more and couldn't explain why," says Brian Wansink, Ph.D., professor of consumer psychology at the University of Illinois, Urbana-Champaign. He goes on to explain that we all look for cues to stop, and in this example, usually that cue is that we've reached the bottom of the popcorn bucket.
- **Watching TV.** Food seems to vanish when we watch TV, read a book, talk on the phone, or surf the Net. Have you ever noticed while watching a suspenseful TV show that the entire bag of pretzels seems to disappear and you don't remember taking a bite? Or, you're so engrossed in a book that you gobble a bag of chocolate chip cookies without even knowing it?

Mindless eating often comes with some interesting subconscious rationalizations. "For some reason, food eaten while I'm standing doesn't count. If I eat it with my fingers, without a fork or spoon, then it really doesn't count. It's unofficial, and in some weird way that means it doesn't have calories," says Anna, a department store salesperson in Chicago, who has been known to nibble her way through an entire apple pie. Food eaten straight from the refrigerator or before you get to the checkout counter also doesn't register. Mindlessly eating off of a partner's plate worked just fine for Dolores as long as the food went directly into her mouth. "I am less likely to eat the sparerib or fry if I put it on my plate instead of directly into my mouth. It's as if the food is calorie-free as long as it doesn't land anywhere," she explains.

Eating on Autopilot: The Downside

It doesn't take a rocket scientist to get the message. Every bite, every mouthful, every taste, every nibble you take—whether you're standing up or sitting down, whether it's on your plate, on your friend's plate, or out of the pan—contains calories. And, no matter what the fad diets tell you about cutting carbs, cutting fat, food combining, or whatnot, the only thing that matters when it comes to battling the bulge is calories. "The growing weight problem in this country is not due to gluttony or a major increase in food intake," says Richard Mattes, Ph.D., R.D., professor of foods and nutrition at Purdue University. "It's due to small energy imbalances, as small as 25 to 100 calories a day, which, over time, build up to a weight problem."

If you're not keeping track of these nibbles, then it's easy to underestimate how much you're eating. You also don't compensate for those extra calories by eating less later. The end result is overeating, usually of all the wrong foods, with your waistline and health taking the brunt of the damage. "All it takes to gain 10 pounds in a year is to consume 100 extra calories every day over and above what you need to maintain a desirable weight," says Moores. That's the calorie equivalent of one big bite of a cheeseburger, a poppy-seed muffin, your child's Halloween candy, or chicken nuggets. The calorie equivalent of four bites of mac and cheese, three bites of birthday cake, or a peanut-butter cup every day also will bump you up a dress size in one year. Worst of all, you didn't even enjoy those bites. You didn't get a thrill from the taste, don't recall the texture, and have no memory of the aroma of a single bite. You've polished off hundreds of calories, and you don't even feel full, let alone satisfied. What a waste! You would be better off skipping all of those mindless, pleasureless bites and saving the calories for a truly delicious treat.

Why is it that we don't nibble mindlessly on broccoli, baby carrots, black beans, wheat germ, or any other real food!? Instead, the foods that typically slide effortlessly into our mouths are greasy, sweet, or both. "If you're going to play the 'one-for-you-and-one-for-me game' with your kids, make sure you're eating blueberries and not a blueberry-flavored yogurt bar dripping with fat and sugar," says Moores, who adds that the blueberries kill two birds with one stone. "You satisfy your hankering to nibble while downing one of the five to eight servings of fruits and vegetables you need every day." The yogurt bar is just empty calories.

Nibbling Is OK

Don't get me wrong—nibbling isn't all bad. It's bad only when we unconsciously nibble our way through the day, falling bite-by-bite further away from our health and weight-loss goals. In contrast, planned and conscious nibbling actually could be the very habit that helps you get back on track.

The nibbler's diet has replaced the "three squares" diet as a better way for a woman to manage her weight, cut her risk for heart disease, and curb her cravings. Researchers at the University of Michigan School of Public Health report that women between the ages of 35 and 69 who divided their food intakes into several little meals and snacks throughout the day were leaner, with less body fat, than were women who ate the same calories but packed them into two or three big meals. In fact, the more little meals and snacks the women ate (up to six a day), the lower their body fat was.

"It makes sense that the body is better adapted to processing small doses of fuel and nutrients all day long than trying to handle a glut of food every so often," says Sharon Edelstein, Sc.M., research scientist at George Washington University and lead researcher on a study that linked snacking with a lower risk for disease. Our ancient ancestors evolved by grazing—not gorging—on nuts, berries, roots, and small game. Feasts were rare and probably occurred only when someone in the tribe slew a woolly mammoth or other large animal. In short, our bodies were designed for nibbling on high-fiber, low-fat foods, not the "gorge-and-fast" eating style of modern society.

Snacking also might help keep the stress hormone cortisol at bay, whereas skipping meals raises stress-hormone levels, which aggravates weight gain by encouraging fat to accumulate around

Nibbling Norms

The little-meals approach to healthy eating has eight guide-posts to keep you on track:

- **Don't take the word *little* lightly.** Eating frequently means budgeting your calories. Limit meals to approximately 500 calories, and limit snacks to 200 calories or fewer, for a daily total of three meals, three snacks, and 1,600 to 2,000 calories.
- **Meals should look good, taste good, and be good for you.** Little meals should be delightful and satisfying (without being satiating) and can even serve as a romantic interlude, while nourishing your body and your soul. Little meals can be as elegant as lemon pasta with asparagus; as earthy as warm, homemade bread with cheese and soup; or as adventuresome as spicy Thai chicken with mangoes.
- **Snacks aren't freebies.** Snacks should contribute to the daily quota of at least eight servings of fruits and vegetables and six servings of whole-grain breads and cereals.

   As a general guideline, include at least one fruit or vegetable and a grain at every snack, and at least two servings of fruits or vegetables and one to two grains at every meal, plus one or more of the following:
   - Nuts and seeds
   - Nonfat milk products, such as milk, yogurt, or cheese
   - Cooked dried beans and peas
   - Extra-lean meats, such as fish, red meat (7 percent fat by weight), or skinless poultry
- **Keep the little-meal plan simple.** Make snacks convenient by having the foods readily available and easy to fix. For example, here are four simple snacks:

- Six ounces of nonfat yogurt sprinkled with sunflower seeds or GrapeNuts
- Fat-free crackers, lean ham slices, and baby carrots
- A fat-free flour tortilla filled with grated zucchini, cheese, and salsa
- Apple slices dipped in cinnamon-apple yogurt
- **Responsible nibbling leaves little or no room for highly processed foods.** Most convenience foods—from commercial cookies, candy, and breakfast bars to chips, flavored popcorn, and "fat-free" desserts—are low in fiber, phytochemicals, vitamins, and minerals. So, opt for the baked potato, not the chips; the orange, not the orange drink; the corn bread, not the corn oil; and the bowl of oatmeal, not the granola bar.
- **Eat often.** During waking hours, allow no more than four hours to pass between little meals or snacks, starting with breakfast.
- **Plan ahead.** Stock your desk drawer, glove compartment, briefcase, or purse with fresh or dried fruit, grains, instant bean soups, fat-free crackers, and other snacks.
- **Eat slowly.** Listen to your body, and eat only enough to leave you comfortably full, not stuffed.

the middle. "Chronic stress jams cortisol into high gear, which increases cravings for foods rich in carbohydrates and fat and encourages any excess calories to be stored in the belly, where they are readily available to fuel the stress response," explains Pamela Peeke, M.D., assistant clinical professor of medicine at the University of Maryland School of Medicine.

The benefits of little meals extend beyond your waistline. David Jenkins, M.D., professor of medicine and nutritional science at the University of Toronto, reports that nibbling lowers blood cholesterol, LDL-cholesterol, and insulin levels and improves insulin sensitivity. "We've noted beneficial changes in blood lipids and insulin levels within weeks of initiating a nibbling style of eating," Jenkins said. He notes that the trickle-down effect on health is a lowered risk of diabetes, heart disease (the number one health concern for women), and possibly even cancers of the colon and breast.

But, wait. Before you start popping more leftovers into your mouth, keep in mind that the secret to snacking is to divide your current food intake into five or six little meals, not to add more food to your usual diet. In other words, have the oatmeal with raisins and orange juice for breakfast, but save the glass of milk and banana for the midmorning snack. Have a sandwich, raw vegetables, and tomato juice for lunch, but save the yogurt and

25 Healthy Nibbles

If you can't resist the urge to nibble, here are a few planned and healthy alternatives to eating that old candy bar stashed in the laundry room.

1. A 2-ounce bran muffin, and half a cantaloupe filled with 6 ounces of low-fat vanilla yogurt
2. An English muffin topped with a thick tomato slice and low-fat cheese, broiled; served with orange juice and fresh blueberries
3. A crepe filled with low-fat ricotta cheese and two pieces of chopped fresh fruit
4. A mix of equal parts of wheat germ, peanut butter, and honey, spread on whole-wheat toast; served with juice or a banana
5. A small container of low-fat yogurt and four graham crackers
6. A cup of warmed, almond-flavored milk and a banana
7. A soft cinnamon pretzel, an apple, and nonfat milk

8. One ounce of sliced turkey, six fat-free crackers, and fresh strawberries
9. Half of a tuna sandwich with a salad (low-fat dressing), tomato slices, and nonfat milk
10. A Greek salad made with feta cheese, cucumbers, tomatoes, and dressing (on the side); served with pita bread, fresh fruit, and nonfat milk
11. A cup of fat-free cottage cheese, fresh fruit, a whole-grain roll or bran muffin, and baby carrots
12. Minestrone soup, bread, a tossed salad, and nonfat milk
13. A whole-wheat raisin bagel topped with 1 tablespoon of fat-free cream cheese and fruit slices
14. A ½ cup of fat-free refried beans with 1 ounce of oven-baked tortilla chips and salsa
15. A cup of low-fat kiwi-strawberry yogurt mixed with two chopped kiwifruits
16. Two slices of whole-wheat toast, each topped with ¼ cup of nonfat cottage cheese and ¼ cup of crushed pineapple
17. A small salad with dressing on the side and a slice of French bread
18. Half of a whole-wheat bagel, toasted and topped with almond butter and a sliced pear
19. Two ounces of salmon on a slice of whole-wheat bread with Dijon mustard
20. A slice of pizza topped with tomato slices
21. A handful of Cherrios (no milk), nuts, and dried fruit
22. Three fig bars and a glass of soy milk
23. A cinnamon-raisin English muffin and fruit
24. A whole-wheat waffle topped with 2 teaspoons of peanut butter and fresh berries
25. A packet of maple and brown sugar instant oatmeal, cooked in nonfat milk and topped with a banana

fruit for the midafternoon snack. Dine on spaghetti, salad, and steamed vegetables in the evening, and then have the slice of French bread and a cup of nonfat cocoa for a late-night snack. The key to weight management and a lifelong healthy diet is eating consciously and purposefully. That means making wise food choices and spreading your food intake evenly throughout the day, starting with breakfast.

Mindful Breakfasts

One reason why some women mindlessly nosh all day could be that they don't start the day off right by eating a nutritious breakfast. "I seldom eat breakfast anymore. Seems like there just isn't enough time in the morning, and I'm not that hungry anyway," says Gloria, a flight attendant in Atlanta.

Big mistake. Breakfast is the most important meal of the day. For most people, the start of the day is the only time that 8, and perhaps 10 or more, hours have gone by between meals. During the hours since dinner, and even while sleeping, the body still needs fuel to keep the normal processes functioning. Much of that fuel comes from readily available stores of glucose. More than half of your glucose reserves are drained by the time morning rolls around, and your body needs a kick start that comes only from a carbohydrate-rich meal.

If you skip breakfast, you still might feel fine, full of energy, and raring to go, for the first few hours after you wake up. That counterfeit burst of energy comes from a mind and body revved from a good night's sleep. However, this initial energy glow wears off for the breakfast skipper as the morning's demands stress a body already running on fumes. By afternoon, even if you eat a relatively good lunch in an effort to boost lagging energy levels, it's too late to acquire the daylong energy you would have had if you'd taken five minutes to eat breakfast. You're also more apt to start eating mindlessly from the refrigerator or your toddler's plate.

Why is breakfast so important to long-term health? One reason is that it may be the most nutritious meal you eat. Today's typical breakfast is high in grains, fruit, and milk, making it a major contributor of vitamins, minerals, and fiber. Gretchen Hill, Ph.D., associate professor in the Department of Animal Science at Michigan State University, studied the effects of breakfast on overall nutrition. She warns, "Women don't catch up on their vitamins, minerals, and fiber—especially vitamin E, zinc, calcium, and iron—missed at breakfast, even if they consume enough calories later in the day." The long-term consequences of these marginal nutrient intakes include chronic fatigue, poor concentration, memory loss, depression, and other physical and mental problems.

Breakfast also helps us stay trim, which reduces the risk for numerous diseases associated with poor health and fatigue, including heart disease, cancer, diabetes, and hypertension. The link between breakfast and a trim figure is threefold:

- Skipping meals slows metabolism, so women who skip breakfast gain weight more readily on fewer calories than do women who eat frequently throughout the day, starting with breakfast.
- Ironically, women actually eat more, not less, when they skip breakfast. "People often think they can save calories by skipping breakfast, but if they kept food journals, they'd find that they more than make up for those saved calories later in the day," says Hill. The brain releases greater amounts of a nerve chemical called neuropeptide Y (NPY) when you skip breakfast, which unconsciously signals you to keep eating. The condition is called "night-eating syndrome": once you start to eat at midday, you don't stop, and you end up consuming more food and calories between noon and bedtime than do people who ate breakfast.
- Breakfast skippers are more prone to mindless eating; they snack throughout the day on less nutritious, high-fat or high-sugar, quick-fix snacks, like chips, candy, and other crispy or sweet snack foods. The overwhelming hunger that comes from the extended fast crushes willpower and leaves a woman so ravenous that she is willing to eat anything as long as it is handy, which can be the leftover waffles on her kid's plate, the

fried dumplings that her honey ordered at the Chinese restaurant, or the chocolate chips right out of the bag. These choices might satisfy immediate hunger, but they fuel fatigue in the long run.

Even if you don't eat more after skipping breakfast, the calories you do eat are more likely to be stockpiled as body fat. A study from Vanderbilt University found that women who ate breakfast lost more weight than did breakfast skippers, even though both groups consumed the same amount of calories. Another study, from the USDA Human Nutrition Research Center, in San Francisco, found that women who ate breakfast while dieting lost more weight than dieters who ate most of their calories later in the day. The National Weight Control Registry

The Breakfast Log

To test the effects of breakfast on your energy level, keep a journal for two or three weeks. (Make copies of the form on page 39, or use it as a guide for designing your own.) Each day, record whether you ate breakfast and, if you did, when you ate and what and how much you had. Don't forget to list coffee—and what you put in it! Then record your food choices, cravings, and energy levels in two- to three-hour increments throughout the day. If you regularly skip breakfast, continue to skip breakfast for the first week of record keeping; then eat a light breakfast during the second week, and note any changes in your mood, energy, and food intake. If you regularly eat breakfast, try skipping this meal for a week and see if you note any changes in how you feel and what you eat. Look for subtle differences on those days when you didn't eat breakfast, such as drinking more coffee at midafternoon or going to bed earlier.

Breakfast Log

On this sheet, record whether you ate breakfast and, if you did, what you had; then record your feelings and food consumption during the day.

Did you eat breakfast? ___ Yes ___ No

If yes, what did you have? _____

	Mood	Food
9 A.M.	_____	_____
11 A.M.	_____	_____
1 P.M.	_____	_____
3 P.M.	_____	_____
5 P.M.	_____	_____
7 P.M.	_____	_____
9 P.M. +	_____	_____

What patterns, if any, did you notice in your mood or food intake for the rest of the day when you ate or skipped breakfast? _____

_____

_____

_____

reports that almost 8 in every 10 people who have lost weight and maintained the weight loss regularly eat breakfast.

Breakfast not only boosts your energy throughout the day, improves exercise performance if you are a morning exerciser, helps you maintain a desirable weight, and keeps you in the top percentile for health—but also prevents mental fatigue. Repeatedly, studies show that people who eat breakfast think better and faster, remember more, react more quickly, and are mentally sharper than breakfast skippers. Perhaps this advantage alone would help you stay alert and less likely to unconsciously nibble or graze!

Compared with breakfast skippers, people who eat breakfast communicate more effectively, make fewer mistakes, complete jobs more quickly, and have better ideas. The effect lasts for up to four hours after eating breakfast.

It's the glucose in the morning meal that revs brainpower. This high-octane fuel enhances learning, memory, and thinking by slowing or preventing the loss of recently acquired information and by enhancing the acquisition and storage of information in the brain. Skip breakfast, and blood levels of lactate, free fatty acids, and beta-hydroxybutyrate increase, which corresponds with poor mental function and reflects the physiological stress placed on the brain when its fuel of choice is missing. The trick to thinking clearly and avoiding mental fatigue is to eat a breakfast that supplies the right type of glucose in the right amount.

Kick the Habit

I hope I've convinced you that mindless eating is a habit you want to remedy and that eating regularly throughout the day, starting with breakfast, is one way to overcome this habit. Just deciding to change or just talking about your eating plans isn't enough. You've got to do some homework if you plan to kick this habit.

Keep a Food Diary

One way to get a grip on what, how much, and when you're eating is to keep a food diary for one week. That's what both the

National Weight Control Registry, an ongoing research study based at Brown University, and Anne Fletcher, M.S., R.D., author of *Thin for Life*, independently found successful dieters do to maintain their weight loss. One trait most of them shared was that they kept food records both during the weight-loss phase and then whenever they noticed even a slight, 5-pound weight regain.

Record keeping isn't a test. There are no right or wrong ways to eat. Record keeping is just a way to increase your awareness of what you're putting into your mouth. "I'm a big advocate of keeping records," says Debra Waterhouse, who likes to call the process "Eat Write." "Keeping records, even for just a few days, brings mindless eating to the mindful level," she adds. The more accurate and honest you are in writing down the foods, the more feedback you'll get on what eating habits you should change and what habits are just fine the way they are. You'll be surprised at what you learn. "You might think you eat only three times a day, but after keeping a food diary, you realize you're eating nonstop," says Waterhouse. One woman said she had no idea how often she grabbed a bite of a cookie or nibbled on desserts left on the kitchen counter until she started keeping a food diary. Those little nibbles seemed so innocent until she added up the calories at the end of the day and found she had eaten more than 400 calories in one-bite snacks.

At the very minimum, you want to record what, how much, and when you eat. If you have the time, also write down how you felt before and after you ate, who else was present or if you were alone, and where you ate the food.

Get out a pad of paper and a pen. Here are the basics of record keeping:

- **Be specific.** Write down everything and in detail. A log that says, "I overate" is too general. A more detailed account would say, "At 11 A.M., I ate 5 tablespoons of rocky road ice cream out of the container while watching a rerun of 'Perry Mason' on TV. Then came back at 11:45 A.M. and had another 4 tablespoons of ice cream with a handful of chocolate chips." This example gives you specific information about the types of food you nibble on, shows that you mindlessly eat while watching TV, and indicates that you are tempted to eat at certain times of the day.

- **Be honest.** Your food records are only as valuable as the information included in them. Don't let guilt get in the way of writing down that bite of your daughter's chocolate Easter bunny nabbed while you were cleaning her room. Write down everything! Many interesting eating patterns pop up only when you've written down everything and kept complete records.
- **Be prompt.** Your recall is best at the moment you are eating. If you wait until later that night or the next day, I promise you will have forgotten half of what you ate.

After a week of record keeping, look back over your diary and see if you find patterns. Just the act of writing everything down may have opened your eyes to how often you pack food into your mouth unknowingly. A simple review of the records may offer other surprises. For example, one woman noticed that she nibbled more doughnuts from the employees' lounge on cool fall mornings. On these mornings, she didn't want to get out of bed and was sleeping later. As a result, she didn't have enough time to eat breakfast, so she was more tempted by the pastries than she was on warmer days when she had eaten before leaving for work. She returned to eating breakfast and was then able to refrain from her doughnut indulgences.

Do I Really Need This?

Mindless nibbling is different for every woman, and so are the ways to get a handle on it. For that reason, a food diary is not for everyone. "For some people, keeping a food record is the best idea for getting a grip on eating patterns, but for others, it's just a burden and they won't do it. For some, it actually backfires because the constant focus on food undoes them," says Richard Mattes. For women who can't or won't keep a food diary, he suggests that they pay closer attention to what they're putting into their mouths: "Mindless eating is not driven by a craving to indulge,

Take a Look at Your Records

The following questions are just a few things to consider when reviewing your records.

- How often am I snatching single bites of food—such as from another person's plate, out of the refrigerator, from leftovers, or out of my child's candy bag?
- What types of foods am I most likely to nibble on: vegetables and other healthful foods or processed, fatty, or sweet treats?
- What cues encourage me to unconsciously graze—for example, the food is in front of me; others are eating; the time of day; the smell of food; a party atmosphere; after a cup of coffee; I'm stressed or feeling grumpy?
- What is my general pattern of eating—three square meals a day; skip meals or eat sporadically; minimeals and snacks evenly distributed; other?
- What am I doing when I eat: is my attention on eating, or am I busy with other projects?
- What excuses or rationales do I use to eat?
- What thoughts or emotions contribute to my nibbling and grazing?
- How do other people influence my decision to eat by their presence, their urgings, or the sight of them eating?
- How much of my food intake is planned, and how much just happens?
- How fast do I eat? What happens when I eat too fast?
- What happens just before I begin nibbling?

and it doesn't satisfy any particular need, so simply asking yourself every time you go to put a bite into you mouth, 'Do I really need this?' may be all it takes to break the habit."

Another approach is to find a focal point during the day when you are most likely to mindlessly eat, and start there. Moores recommends focusing on what you do before and after each meal. "Often I find that when a woman can tie her attention to some routine event, such as dinner, she has an easier time identifying habits that are undermining her best intentions to eat well," she says. Try paying extra-close attention to your eating while you're preparing meals and during cleanup. Do you repeatedly taste-test, nibble on munchies, or drink wine while cooking? Or, are you the cleanup queen, putting leftovers into your mouth rather than down the disposal? Look for little, subtle ways in which you tend to take in extra calories beyond just what makes it to your plate.

Once you identify—from your food records or just from becoming more aware of your eating style—what habits are getting in your way of becoming leaner or being the healthiest you can be, you can develop a plan for making changes to create a new habit.

Choose a New Habit

The good news about changing this habit of mindless eating is that it probably won't take a huge amount of effort. "The best way to make sustainable changes in your eating habits that will result in a healthier and maybe leaner you is to keep those changes small, such as not eating the leftovers as you clean the kitchen. This small step doesn't require any major changes in how or what you eat, but it could result in significant health benefits over the long run," says Mattes.

Be with Your Food

The most obvious way to stop eating mindlessly is to *eat only when you are paying attention*, preferably only at planned meals and snacks. Nothing goes into your mouth, other than water, at any other time. Debra Waterhouse recommends that before you eat, you remind yourself to look at the food, take in the aromas, and then slowly eat the first two bites. "This simple exercise really helps you pay attention to something you often do unconsciously," she says. Or, ask yourself, "How often do I sit when I am eating?" If your answer is never, that's a good indication that you need to establish a designated spot where you sit down to eat, and eat only there. Don't eat out of the container, box, or bag. Instead, serve yourself a portion on a plate, carry it to the table, take a deep breath, and learn what eating mindfully feels like. I promise that you will enjoy the flavors, aromas, and textures of food much more when you are paying attention. You also may find that you eat less, and more healthfully.

Create Solutions from Your Records

You'll find all kinds of ideas for how to nip mindless eating in the bud just by looking over your food records. For example, the kitchen is a prime target for inhaling invisible calories. Rather than consuming the calorie equivalent of a full dinner before even sitting down to a meal, try chewing gum or drinking ice water while cooking. Or munch on something low-calorie and healthy. For example, snacking on baby carrots or apple slices is a much better option than finishing off the bag of chips while you're cooking. Besides, no one will ever holler at you for eating too many fruits or vegetables!

When it comes to grazing after a meal, Moores recommends, "You might choose to have someone else in the family clean up the kitchen, so you aren't tempted by the leftovers, or have someone help you with cleanup so that you chat, rather than eat." Or, you could give the leftovers to a friend to take home. If all else fails, put leftovers in the garbage or down the disposal; leave the dishes until morning, when the food won't be as appetizing; or drown all plates and pots in the sink. Be creative in finding solutions to your mindless-eating dilemmas.

If you eat from others' plates, both inside and outside the home, then you might choose to eat only food that is portioned on your plate. "You're better off deciding what you want to eat and then putting a serving on a plate," says Barbara Rolls, Ph.D., professor of nutrition at Pennsylvania State University. "That way, you get the full range of information on how much you're eating and are less likely to overdo it." That means no nibbling from the container, at the serving platter, while cooking, or off of the kids' or your spouse's plates!

Eat Consistently, Not Constantly

Wayne C. Callaway, M.D., former associate clinical professor of medicine at George Washington University, recommends establishing a consistent pattern of eating, which, over the course of a few weeks, will help reprogram your body's appetite and hunger clock. Take a long look at your food records to review what and how you are eating. "You're looking not only for the types of foods you choose but also for how you distribute that food throughout the day," says Callaway. Meal skippers are most prone to consume grab-and-go food throughout the day and then overindulge later in the afternoon or evening. In this case, you should redistribute your food by eating a nutritious breakfast, taking snacks along with you to eat when you are comfortably hungry during the day, and then eating a moderate dinner. No nibbling in between these meals.

Eat Breakfast

If your records show that the cause of your relentless nibbling is that you are a seasoned breakfast-avoider, then start eating breakfast, even if you are not hungry. "It takes two to three weeks to reset the appetite clock," says Callaway. After that, you should notice a gain in energy and mental power, if you're choosing the correct foods. Avoid high-sugar breakfasts, such as doughnuts and coffee; they provide an initial energy boost but leave you drowsy within a few hours. The best energy-boosting breakfasts are ones that are light and healthful and that mix a little protein, such as mik or peanut butter, with even more carbohydrates, such as cereal, toast, or low-fat waffles.

Researchers at the Institute of Food Research, in Redding, England, report that eating breakfast helps you feel more upbeat if that breakfast is mostly grains and fruit. In their study, 16 people answered questionnaires about their moods and took tests measuring their memories before and after eating either low-fat/high-carbohydrate or high-fat/low-carbohydrate breakfasts. Those people who ate the low-fat/high-carbohydrate breakfasts reported feeling more cheerful and more energetic for at least two and a half hours. In contrast, high-fat or big breakfasts slow you down and muddle thinking.

Combining a little protein with the carbohydrates at breakfast helps keep you full and energized throughout the morning hours, so you are less likely to finish off the last bites of your child's Happy Meal. A study from the Wageningen Agricultural University, in Holland, found that planning breakfast around carbohydrates with small amounts of protein reduced hunger throughout the morning, while high-fat, protein-laden breakfasts, such as eggs and bacon, led to overeating at lunchtime. A bowl of carbohydrate-rich cereal topped with low-fat milk should keep you energized throughout most of the day, while a high-fat, high-protein breakfast of steak and eggs or a cheese omelet could leave you longing for a nap. Make sure that the carbohydrate comes packaged with fiber by choosing whole—not refined—grains, and you'll feel full longer and be less likely to eat sugary foods later in the day.

The best news is that healthful, light breakfasts also are the easiest to prepare. Whether you have been a breakfast skipper or you eat breakfast every day, there is no reason to add stress to your morning routine by trying to fix elaborate, time-intensive breakfasts, especially when it shouldn't take more than five minutes to prepare everything you need to fuel yourself through the morning hours.

Mindful Eating

There are more benefits to breaking the mindless-eating habit than just physical health or losing a few pounds. Food is more than just what you eat. It's also about how and with whom you eat. "Eating mindfully and with gratitude—that is, eating not only *for* the heart but also *from* the heart—affects how well food is metabolized and used in the body," says Deborah Kesten,

Breakfast Guidelines: As Simple as 1, 2, 3

A typical healthy breakfast takes only five minutes to prepare and is as simple as a bowl of cereal with low-fat milk and a tall glass of orange juice. Here are the guidelines:

1. Include two servings of fruits (or vegetables) from the following list:
   - Six ounces of 100 percent fruit or vegetable juice (Avoid all juices made with pear, white grape, or apple juice concentrate, since these "all-natural" fruit beverages are actually primarily sugar water. Instead, choose 100 percent orange juice, grapefruit juice, orange-pineapple juice, or tomato juice, or fresh-squeeze your own juices if you have time.)
   - A piece of fruit, such as a plum, pear, apple, banana, orange, papaya (half), peach, tangerine, grapefruit, or kiwifruit, or 1 cup of cantaloupe or other melon.
   - Dried fruit—2 tablespoons or more
2. Select one to three servings of a high-carbohydrate, high-fiber food from the following list:
   - A slice of whole-wheat bread, half of a whole-wheat bagel or English muffin, a whole-wheat flour tortilla, or a low-fat whole-wheat scone
   - A low-fat muffin, preferably whole wheat, bran, carrot, or fruit-filled
   - A slice of corn bread
   - One to 2 ounces of ready-to-eat cereal
   - ½ cup of cooked whole-grain hot cereal, such as oatmeal, multigrain cereal, or wheat germ

3. Select one serving of a protein-rich food from the following list:
   - Fat-free or low-fat milk or yogurt (1 cup), cottage cheese (2 cups), cheese (1 ounce), or ricotta cheese (2 ounces)
   - A thin slice of meat, such as turkey, chicken, or beef (1 to 3 ounces)
   - Peanut or almond butter (2 tablespoons), cooked dried beans (1 cup), or tofu (3 to 4 ounces)
   - ¼ to ½ cup of egg substitute, one whole egg, or two egg whites

M.P.H., a pioneer in the field of integrative nutrition and the author of *The Healing Secrets of Foods*. Kesten believes food is most healthful when consumed in a peaceful environment, at a calm pace, and with enjoyable company. In contrast, wolfing food, eating when stressed or angry, and bickering at the table are all experiences associated with increased risk factors for disease and ill health. "What you eat is certainly important," says Kesten, "but how and with whom you eat are also essential to your physical and mental health, as well as to the nourishment of your soul."

Slowing the pace and eating mindfully worked for Laura. She confides: "Unconscious eating was just one symptom of how my life had become too hectic. Once I started slowing down and paying attention to what I ate, I found I became more aware of my life in general. Now I choose only foods that nourish me, and I've stopped shoveling the kids' leftovers into my mouth just because they are there. I've lost the weight, but more important, I feel great and more in control of my eating."

Putting Others' Needs Ahead of Our Own

When I met my future husband, I was a vegetarian from California, and he was a "pork roast, mashed potatoes, and gravy" man from the Midwest. He expected me to cook, but when I prepared tofu stir-fry, salads, and roasted-vegetable burritos, he hovered over my shoulder, making suggestions and complaining. The tension mounted until I eventually started eating fish and chicken and learned to tolerate junk food in the house. Then the kids came along, and the ginger-glazed salmon and spicy enchiladas were replaced with macaroni and cheese, fat-free hot dogs, and pizza. I couldn't even prepare chicken breast without the kids' complaining that it was too dry and hard to chew. My diet slowly changed, and finding time for exercise became an increasing challenge as I accommodated the family's needs.

My story is not unusual. Women are famous for putting others' needs before their own. We make the best (not perfect) food choices when we are on our own. Put us into relationships with partners, family, friends, or children, and we eat and drink more, choose ribs or tater tots instead of salads, and consume more calories, fat, and sugar.

The temptation to be sidetracked from our diet goals goes beyond just family and friends. It's all around us. Kelly Brownell, Ph.D., professor of psychology at Yale University, calls our society a "toxic environment." According to

Brownell, "We are exposed to an unprecedented supply of poor-quality food that is widely available, low-cost, heavily promoted, and great-tasting." In one survey, too much temptation and pressure to eat high-calorie foods was the number one obstacle to eating well for 43 percent of women.

Caving in to these pressures and to others' preferences and demands can happen anytime, anywhere, and with anyone. However, there are five classic situations in which many women are tempted to stray from their best intentions to eat sensibly. These are getting married, caring for children, attending family get-togethers, socializing with friends, and dining out.

Love 'n' Marriage: Together in Eating

While the bride-to-be might resort to near starvation to reach fighting weight for the big day, once the wedding bells toll, eating begins. Swap the social scene for home life, and there are more nights sitting around the tube, more food at your fingertips, more alcohol, less time at the gym, and a little less concern about watching every calorie. "Compared with the way I spent my time when single, now that I'm married, we spend more evenings eating out, at the movies with a bag of popcorn, or sharing a sundae at the ice cream parlor. I'm comfortable with my man, so it's not as big a deal if I put on a little weight," says Tricia, a magazine editor in Los Angeles. In fact, some women gain 6 to 8 pounds in the first two years of marriage and average 25 pounds in the first 13 years of marriage. Unhappily married women gain 42 pounds (for more on how we turn to food to sooth our moods, see Habit 7: I'm Moody—Let's Eat!). According to a study from Cornell University, newlyweds gain more weight than do singles or people who are widowed or divorced.

"One reason for postwedding weight gain is that women lose their dietary independence," says Edward Abramson, Ph.D., professor emeritus at California State University at Chico and author of *Body Intelligence*. "Before marriage, when a roommate fantasized about meat loaf and gravy for dinner, a woman might respond by saying, 'That's fine; make it yourself.' Now she is blending her nutritional needs with a partner, and more often than not, she is the one expected to cook." The fact that 8 out of every 10 women are the primary household food shoppers attests to the role women play as gatekeepers and family food managers of this nation's home-cooked meals! Combine a budding relationship with repeated exposure to buying and preparing food, and you have the perfect opportunity for weight gain.

We also consume more when we eat in tandem than when we eat alone. We might be content with a 350-calorie Lean Cuisine entree and a salad when munching solo, but share a meal with a partner and the calories soar two- to threefold. We linger over the meal longer, eat foods we wouldn't eat otherwise, and drink more. Having a buddy there makes it acceptable and fun to indulge in more sinful foods, such as cookies, chips, and fries. "A single woman often spends a lot of energy dieting in order to stay in the dating game. Once married, it's hard to maintain that effort," says Abramson. The subtle, often unconscious "I've got him now, so I don't have to work so hard" mentality can lead to a gradual relaxing of the diet guard. Succumbing night after night, week after week, month after month, for years means many women pack on a little extra weight or slip from their plans to eat healthfully.

Men Can Get Away with Eating More; We Can't

People, in general, tend to adopt a loved one's eating habits. For women, that means more meat, gravy, and pizza, and less salad. Jeffrey Sobal, Ph.D., of Cornell University, says, "Think about it—you're going to be eating with this person for the rest of your life. You'd probably be most comfortable with someone who shares your individual eating habits." How likely is *that*? Instead, many of us, like myself, wind up in the kitchen with a partner whose eating habits are as alien from ours as Mars is from Venus.

It's not that men are out to get us; it's just that their eating habits are very different. For one thing, they can eat more without having the calories go to their hips and thighs. "Say a woman finishes her dinner, but her partner is still eating. It's rude to leave him at the table alone, so the woman keeps him company, and while they chat, she nibbles from the serving bowl or heaps

another helping onto her plate," says Abramson. Even a sedentary man can munch up to 2,900 calories a day without gaining
an ounce, while that man's couch-potato wife might gain weight
on as few as 1,600 calories. Because of this calorie gap, men can
afford to waste calories on junk and still meet their nutritional
needs, while every morsel counts for a woman.

In general, men gravitate to the high-fat meats, beer, and
liquor, while shunning the low-calorie and fiber-rich vegetables,
fruits, and whole grains. A spinach salad with black beans and
low-fat cheese satisfies a woman's need for protein, folic acid, and
calcium without the calories, but many husbands would say that
a salad isn't a meal and that it is certainly not a meal if it doesn't
contain meat. Yet, if a woman eats like a man, she'll stack the deck
in favor of gaining weight and clogging her arteries. In short,
equality might be fine for most areas of a marriage, but have what
he's having, and wham, you'll gain weight faster than you can say
"pepperoni pizza with extra cheese, please."

The inequality of the sexes is most pronounced at restaurants.
"Before the kids were born, my husband and I loved to go out to
eat where we could catch up on our day without the distractions
of home," says LeAnn, a dental hygienist in Columbus. She often
ordered the same foods as her husband, or foods she never would
have dreamed of eating at home, such as a steak and fries or crispy
chicken. As a result, she put on 7 pounds during that first year
of marriage. Do the math, and you'll see how easy it is to put on
weight. Have an order of chicken nuggets instead of a grilled-
chicken salad, and you're consuming 300 extra calories. Do that
day after day, and those extra calories equate to a 31-pound
weight gain in one year! Granted, we don't gobble that many extra
calories every day, but doing it even once a week can mean 4 extra
pounds by year's end.

Whose Side Is He On?

For many women, when the weight creeps up and they decide to
do something about it, they don't get the support from their
mates that they expected. In one study, 9 out of 10 women seek-

ing help from obesity experts stated that sabotage was a major obstacle to their efforts.

"There are a variety of reasons why some husbands try to undermine their partner's attempt to lose weight," says Abramson. A man might anticipate that if his wife gives up ice cream or chips and gets fit, he will be expected to do the same. As long as she is overweight, it's all right that he's fat, too. "The trade-off factor is a common reason for sabotage," says Abramson, who cites the example of a husband who has a problem with drinking, gambling, or smoking and feels that as long as his wife is unsuccessful at weight loss, he won't be expected to quit his habit. "Then there is the chastity-belt phenomenon, where her love handles have been his excuse for their dismal love life, or he fears that if she loses the weight, he won't be good enough for her anymore." In other words, he might sabotage her efforts in order to avoid confronting deeper or more personal, uncomfortable issues. You know you've got a sabotage issue on your hands if:

- Instead of praising the Cajun salmon salad, he complains that it's not pork roast and gravy.
- He grumbles that you're not buying all the goodies he is used to having in the house.
- He offers to do the grocery shopping and brings home lots of tempting foods not on your meal plan.
- Rather than walk with you after dinner, he brings home a box of chocolates to reward your efforts.
- He complains that he's lonely when you leave the house to exercise.
- He gripes about the cost of your gym membership, aerobic classes, or exercise equipment.
- He surprises you with KFC after you ban fried foods from the house.
- When all else fails, he becomes sullen and angry for no apparent reason.

A hefty support team is crucial to sticking with a healthy eating plan, as well as shedding pounds and keeping them off.

Research shows that women are most successful at maintaining nutritious eating habits when their partners participate in their diet and exercise routines. In one study, women were three times more likely to stick with a weight-loss program and lost 35 percent more weight when they joined the program with their hubbies than when they signed up solo. People also are most likely to follow healthy diet plans that lower their risk for diseases, such as heart disease, if they can count on encouragement from loved ones.

Babies and Weight Gain

Women face an even greater challenge when the kids arrive. Ask any mother, and she'll tell you it was a lot easier to maintain her girlish figure before she had sleepless nights, irregular feeding schedules, no time to exercise, and a ready supply of Ding Dongs, Ho Hos, and Cheez Whiz in the house. According to a study from Duke University, women face a 7 percent increased risk for weight problems with every child. On the other hand, a baby in the house has only a mild effect on a man's risk for weight gain. "My life since the kids were born is a job of juggling marriage, children, my career, time for exercise, and volunteer work, with my biggest priorities being my family and job. That means my own health often takes a backseat," says Monique, an elementary school teacher and the mother of two preschool children in Orlando. Many times, these women do the minimum for themselves. Aside from on-again, off-again attempts at dieting, nutrition often winds up at the back of the bus for working mothers.

As discussed in the previous chapter, mothers nibble on their children's leftovers while cleaning the kitchen and in a one-bite-for-you-and-one-bite-for-me style. Every bite means extra calories. We also tend to eat even if we're not hungry if there are kids around. "Dinner is the only meal that I eat with my kids during the week," says Jennifer, a working mom in Cincinnati, "so, I feel as if I have to eat with them, even if I'm not hungry." Sue, a graphic artist outside Boston, would fix the children their dinner in the early evening and would end up eating with them. "Then," she recounts, "my husband came home at eight-thirty or nine, and I'd have a glass of wine and a second dinner with him." As a result, her pants had inched up two sizes in six years.

Mealtime Peer Pressure

Even if you aren't married with children, you might be tempted to overeat when you're out with friends or dining with family members. For example, your friend says casually, "I'm famished." Whereas a moment before, food was the last thing on your mind, now you're hungry, too. "Nowhere is the power of suggestion stronger than when it comes to food," says Susan Moores, M.S., R.D., spokesperson for the American Dietetic Association. One study from the University of Toronto found that people were most likely to say they were hungry when told that others who had been in the same room before them had been extremely hungry. Not only is hunger catching, but also, the greater the number of people around, the hungrier you're likely to become and the more food you're likely to eat, especially if your meal buddies love to eat.

Family pressure can be the most daunting. A mother-in-law who lays on the guilt to coerce you into having one more piece of chocolate cake or a father who says you are too skinny and drops another dollop of mashed potatoes on your plate can be someone to whom it is difficult to "just say no." Stephanie, a public relations account executive in Atlanta, can attest to that: "Every time I go to my mother-in-law's house, and no matter how hard I try, I always eat too much. My resolve seems to melt when someone asks me to try the meatballs or any other appetizer. A glass of wine and any remaining willpower flies out the window. Once I start nibbling, I can't stop and have been known to polish off a tray of crab puffs." Michelle, an attorney in Northern California, confesses, "I'm a sucker for a little coaxing. My mother makes the best candied sweet potatoes. I start out having a small scoop, but all it takes is for her to plead with me to have another serving, and there I am scooping a second generous pile onto my plate."

Friends and family can be expert saboteurs. Maybe your sister is uncomfortable eating in front of you or is jealous of your success. Maybe a good friend doesn't want you to succeed or wants to test your resolve, so she tempts or teases you to see how serious you are. A cousin pressures you when standing in front of the cinnamon roll shop at the mall, by saying, "I'll have one if you'll have one," or "Come on, just split one with me," or "You've been so good on your diet, you deserve to treat yourself. Besides, half of mine isn't so bad." It might not be deliberate sabotage; your tempter might just need absolution from her own eating "sins." Of course, issues such as those are the other person's problem, and you shouldn't let it become yours by agreeing to eat, but sometimes it might seem easier to give in than to hold the fort.

Holidays are the supreme example of family pressure run amok. Let's face it. Starting at Thanksgiving and continuing through New Year's Day, you are constantly tempted by the most enticing treats under your most vulnerable circumstances. You may dodge the fudge at the office party, only to succumb to your mother's plea to have one more piece of homemade pumpkin cheesecake. You might gracefully say no to the butter cookies offered at a neighbor's house, only to be slipped a candy cane by a department-store Santa. Then there's the guests coming over, the dinner parties at friends' houses, and the daily treats at the office. "I have eaten a whole lot of stuff at holidays just so that I would be accepted," says Valerie, an airport security manager in Portland, Oregon. "I even ate lamb at Easter, and I hate lamb!" Sometimes it seems that the holidays exist just to see how much temptation a woman can handle! It's no wonder we average a 1- to 2-pound weight gain during the holiday season, which equates to an extra 7,000 calories' worth of eggnog, hors d'oeuvres, and home cooking. Never fear. Mastering a few simple tricks discussed later in this chapter is all it takes to resist temptation and pressure from loved ones.

Dining Out Can Do Us In

Then there is the issue of socializing at restaurants where menus and servers entice us to eat more than we want. Never before in the history of the planet have we dined out as often as we do today. "When I was a kid, going to a restaurant was a special occasion. We kids got to order whatever we wanted—within reason, of course—and I always asked for extra fries," says Helen, an emergency-room nurse in San Francisco. Eating out was once a treat, but now it's a routine, with one in every five meals eaten at a restaurant, for a total of more than 53 billion meals and almost $300 billion per year, according to the National Restaurant Association. Almost 1 in 10 women eats out up to seven times a week! More than 45 percent of money spent on food goes to restaurant meals and other away-from-home foods today, up from 34 percent in 1970.

The more we eat out, the less nutritious our diets become. Many of us still adopt the "treat" mentality of long ago, so we are less likely to question the calories or healthfulness of a meal and are more likely to indulge in gooey or greasy dishes that we wouldn't dream of eating at home. We use excuses like, "I'm paying for it, so I might as well finish it," "Just this once won't hurt," "I hate to waste food," or "Poor me—I deserve a treat." While we might pinch and scrimp on every extra calorie at home, we turn a blind eye to platters of mysterious foods served by strangers at a restaurant, never considering the calorie consequences. That mentality gets us into trouble, since restaurant meals are typically much higher in calories and fat than home-cooked foods. Those meals also are typically higher in saturated fat and lower in fiber, calcium, and iron, because they are sorely lacking in colorful produce, whole grains, nonfat milk or soy milk, and legumes.

Fast-food restaurants are the worst. In an effort to edge out the competition, the drive-through offers ever-bigger, megasize servings. These "value meals" are extra-heavy on the fat and calories. Don't be fooled by those fast-food salads, either. They might sound healthy, but they often are just a burger in a bowl, packing in the same amount of fat and calories as a Quarter Pounder with Cheese, and sometimes more. Take, for example, a McDonald's Crispy Chicken Bacon Ranch Salad with dressing, which contains 640 calories and 12 teaspoons of fat, more than a Big Mac. It's no surprise that a woman's risk for weight problems increases with the number of times per week she dines out.

Kick the Habit

In the Introduction, you learned what to eat to be healthy and svelte. Now it's time to learn how to stick with that plan, no matter who or what tempts you otherwise. The golden rule of healthy eating is to eat only when you are truly hungry, not because someone offers you food, wants your company while eating, orders it at a restaurant, or is eating in front of you. Then stop when you are comfortably full, not stuffed.

Eating only when truly hungry means getting back in touch with your body's natural ability to monitor food intake. Start listening to your body. Tune in to your natural hunger signals, making a distinction between stomach hunger (true hunger symptoms include an emptiness in your stomach and stomach rumblings) and social hunger (eating because the food is there or because someone wants you to eat it). If you are truly hungry, don't deny yourself. Ask yourself, "What would satisfy this particular hunger?" Then eat what seems like a good match, not because someone offers it to you or tempts or pressures you to eat. In addition, eat mindfully. Pay attention to and enjoy every mouthful. Then stop halfway through the meal, sit back, and pay attention to your body. If you still feel physically hungry, have another few bites, stop, and listen again. Stop when you are comfortably full, and say no to the offers for seconds or a piece of pie.

The Plan: Set Limits

OK. So, you've checked your stomach hunger and you know you don't want another bite. How do you resist temptation? How do you stick with your plan to eat well in spite of a family who demands pizza and ice cream? How do you enjoy family gatherings without stuffing yourself on food that you don't even want? How do you dine out without gobbling a platter, instead of a plate, of food?

The first step to resisting temptation is to become aware of how others influence your eating habits. For one week, monitor your interaction with others when there is food around. Don't judge. Don't criticize. Just observe with a "Hmmm, that's interesting" attitude. You probably will notice patterns, and from that information, you can proceed to the second step, which is to develop a plan.

Whether it's at home with your partner or children, at family gatherings, or with friends at a restaurant, the eating situation needs to be approached with specific strategies that are part of a plan you create for how you will respond to food offers, social pressure, or temptations to eat too much. Use the work sheet, "My Plan to Fend Off Pressures to Eat," at the end of this chapter to create strategies that will work best for you. For example:

- At home with your partner, you might plan to eat slowly to give yourself more time to recognize when you're still hungry and when you are full. Another possible tactic is to take your plate and silverware to the kitchen once you're done so that you're not tempted to have a second helping or to nibble off of his plate.
- Make a contract with your partner in which you agree not to give each other food gifts or not to use food as entertainment. Visit a museum or play miniature golf instead of going out for ice cream when you need to get out of the house. Or, create rituals that don't involve food; read a book to each other rather than gorge on pizza on Friday night.
- Set a limit on nibbling off of the children's plates: no more than two bites of a child's meal, and only after the child is done.
- Anticipate pressures from family members to eat. Practice what you will say ahead of time to deflect these temptations.
- Before you arrive at a restaurant, make the decision that you will ask for foods grilled without fat, remove the bread and butter from the table, and avoid high-fat add-ons to salads, such as sour cream, cheese, croutons, bacon bits, and full-fat dressing.

Tell It Like It Is

A huge part of your plan to resist temptation is effective communication. You need to speak up, listen, and model the behaviors you want to encourage in others.

- **Speak up.** Ask for cooperation. Be willing to say no and stick to it. Speak your mind in a polite, but firm, way so that both your body language and your words clearly communicate your resolve. Regardless of the reason, refuse food you don't want, and continue to refuse until others get the message. You needn't be confrontational; just gently and politely say, "No, thank you." You might respond to a friend who refuses to take no for an answer to her offer of a second helping by saying, "No, thanks; I would love to have more, but I'm full" or "It was delicious, but I have already had plenty." When your spouse wants to stop for a milkshake, say, "You go ahead, but I don't want the extra calories."

  Your spouse and children are likely to be especially concerned about how your desire to eat well will affect them. Discuss what impact it might have on their lives, and brainstorm solutions so that everyone is satisfied. If the entire household gets on board with your healthy eating plan, the likelihood of your reaching your health or weight-loss goals is much greater.

  Besides feeling threatened or jealous, some people equate eating healthy with starvation. So, reassure the gang that you are eating well and are satisfying your hunger and your body's needs. If friends or family tease you about your efforts to eat well, don't let them distract you from your goals. Stand firm and remind them how serious you are about making these nutrition changes. Politely suggest to family and friends that restaurants with healthy choices be selected when you're planning on dining out. Be on guard. Sabotage can come in subtle forms, such as a friend who says you have lost enough weight or have eaten enough vegetables today, so you now have the right to splurge. Be positive. Be upbeat. But, be firm.

- **Listen.** Communication is a two-way street. That means you need to honestly and openly share your feelings, *and* you need to listen to others' thoughts. People are more apt to listen to you and to understand your needs if they feel you have listened to them. That means paying attention to both verbal and nonverbal signals and sometimes repeating what you think the person is saying to make sure you got it right. As mentioned previously, there are lots of reasons why loved ones sabotage your best efforts to eat well. Understanding each other is a prerequisite to gaining the support you need from people to stick with a healthful eating plan.

Understanding begins with listening. For example, if your spouse is angry or anxious because he fears your changes will mean changes for him, too, use this occasion as the starting ground for finding a plan or compromise that will work for both of you. Maybe you agree to fix him his favorite meal once or twice a week, instead of every night. Or, he cooks and you make the salad (an added benefit here is that you share time together while preparing the meal). Ask loved ones who resist your new eating plan to explain what they are feeling and thinking. An essential way to encourage support and resolve problems is to reassure loved ones who feel threatened by your efforts and to talk openly and honestly about the situation.

- **Set an example.** People are most likely to understand the type of support you need if they are given an example. Display the type of support you want for your efforts by complimenting others on their successes and acting like the friend you want to have.

Are You Part of the Problem?

It is important to make sure you're not contributing to the sabotage. Beliefs you hold and assumptions you make can lead you to feel obligated to eat, just as Valerie felt obligated to eat lamb on Easter. When a coworker brings you homemade fudge, do you feel it isn't right to refuse a gift, even though fudge is not part of your new eating plan? If so, you might allow yourself to be sabotaged. You will have a difficult time handling social pressures if you worry that you'll hurt someone's feelings if you refuse food. The solution here is to change any beliefs that are interfering with

Am I Sabotaging Myself? A Quiz

Sometimes our beliefs, assumptions, and excuses leave us vulnerable to sabotage. Rate yourself on the following statements, and then total your score.

1 = Strongly disagree
2 = Agree
3 = Strongly agree

___ 1. I should eat if someone else is paying for it.

___ 2. It isn't right to refuse food when someone has made or bought it for me.

___ 3. I'd rather give in to someone else's request than hurt the person's feelings.

___ 4. I have to eat when I see others eating.

___ 5. I feel guilty changing if someone I love doesn't want me to change.

___ 6. Other people need or depend on me, and their needs are more important than mine.

___ 7. It's not nice to refuse or say no when someone is just trying to be nice or helpful.

___ 8. I can't stand up and speak my mind or ask for what I need or want.

___ 9. It's my decision to change my eating habits, so it's not fair that I ask others to help me.

___ 10. If you invite people to dinner, you should serve them fancy meals, which are high in fat or calories.

___ 11. I can't resist food or beverages when I'm at a party or social event.

___ 12. I would be imposing and making a nuisance of myself if I asked a hostess to make something special for me or if it would be all right to bring a dish, so I can't do it.

___ 13. I shouldn't involve other people in my problems and dieting efforts.

___ 14. When eating in a restaurant, I should clean my plate, because I'm paying for it.

Scoring:

25 to 42: Saboteur. You are a major player in sabotaging your diet efforts. Your beliefs, assumptions, and excuses are getting in your way of getting on with your health. Start today to change your belief system so that it will encourage, rather than undermine, your attempts to eat well or lose weight.

17 to 24: Accomplice. Your beliefs and assumptions often get in the way of your diet efforts. Changing even a few beliefs could make a big difference in your success.

Less than 17: Resistor. Congratulations. You have developed a healthy belief system that will aid your efforts regarding health and weight management.

your efforts and then to openly and honestly communicate what you want and need from others, so that they can help support your health and weight-loss efforts. The beliefs and rationales we use that get in our way are discussed in detail in Habit 6: Excuses, Excuses, Excuses.

Eating Well at Home

Being married with kids is not a ticket to weight gain. In fact, guys and kids aren't necessarily all that opposed to healthy meals. "Most men want to eat well and take good care of themselves," says Ken Druck, Ph.D., author of *The Secrets Men Keep*, "but

they've inherited an age-old belief that dieting means deprivation." The most important thing to remember is that your husband's health is ultimately his responsibility—not yours. When
it comes to kids, it is your responsibility to stock the kitchen and
serve healthy meals; it's their responsibility to choose from those
selections (that is, you can offer brussels sprouts, but you can't
force children to eat them). Don't set yourself up for disappoint-
ment or anger when your son ignores your advice or when your
daughter turns up her nose at your tofu burgers or spinach salad.
Eventually they'll come around. The following suggestions will
help speed the process.

Set Realistic Goals. Don't expect husbands and kids to go from
loving burgers to craving broccoli overnight. Nutrition is rarely
high on their agenda, so plan for the process to take months, even
years. "We hold tightly to our food habits, perhaps because we
practice them daily," says Mary Donkersloot, R.D., a nutrition
therapist in Beverly Hills. As a result, she says, "Making even simple changes can seem monumental." Every two to three months,
set a new minigoal, such as switching from 2 percent milk to
skim, or from regular to low-calorie salad dressing. Over the long
haul, these small changes will make a huge difference in your and
your family's overall health.

Emphasize the Positive. Faced with a major health problem,
such as skyrocketing cholesterol levels, a man is likely to ponder
ordering fillet of sole instead of filet mignon. Unfortunately, fear
is a short-term motivator. Eventually it'll create an attitude of "I'm
doomed anyway; I might as well have steak." So, don't expect him
to jump onto your support wagon if you tell him he'll die if he
keeps eating poorly. A better approach is to point out that he can
improve his health by supporting your desire to make better
choices. For instance, don't say that french fries will kill him;
instead, suggest he try your baked sweet-potato fries, because they
contain a lot of beta-carotene, which will reduce his risk of cancer (at the same time, they are trimming your waistline and
improving your health, too!).

Lose the Attitude. "You can undermine best intentions to revamp your family's eating habits if you present a tasty, healthful meal with a 'holier-than-thou' attitude," says Druck. Leave your judgments and opinions at the door, and come to the table with an open, accepting manner.

Stock Up. You and your family are most likely to eat nutritious food if it's available. Fill the fridge with easy-to-grab, healthy snacks that fit with your new eating plan. When family members prowl the kitchen, they'll surface with fresh fruit (already cut up), dried fruit, frozen grapes, and whole-wheat crackers. Leftovers are a man's best friend, so make sure there's always a little extra from last night's nutritious meal. He might learn to love that low-fat vegetable-beef soup if he tries it often enough. (For tips on how to shop and stock the kitchen with healthful additions, see Habit 5: Setting Off Without a Plan.)

Revamp Favorite Foods. As you explore the no-man's-land between your nutritional needs and your family's food preferences, you might find some common ground. "It's amazing what you can do with ground turkey breast," says Evelyn Tribole, R.D., author of *Stealth Health: How to Sneak Nutrition Painlessly into Your Diet*. Tribole uses half ground turkey and half extra-lean ground beef when making chili. "No one even knows the difference," she says.

Cut Portions. Some partners are set in their eating ways and simply refuse to give up their favorite foods. In this case, cook the desired foods, but make less. "Even a 6-ounce steak is better than a 12-once one," says Brenda Ponichtera, R.D., author of *Quick and Healthy: Recipes and Ideas for People Who Say They Don't Have Time to Cook Healthy Meals*. Then serve yourself a 3-ounce portion, and make up the difference with extra vegetables and salads that will fill you up without filling you out.

Disguise Healthy Foods. "The problem food at our house is broccoli, so I add it to my pesto sauce," says Tribole. "It's green

Favorite Family-Food Makeovers

Many of your family's favorite foods, such as steak, gravy, and meat loaf, are right up there with Mom and apple pie as all-American symbols. Too bad they are also icons for an unhealthy diet. They don't have to be. Try these slimmed-down versions of four best-loved foods. You will improve your health without sacrificing your family's taste buds.

- **Cheeseburgers:** Make small hamburgers using a 50-50 mixture of ground turkey breast and ground sirloin (7 percent fat or less by weight). Top with leaf (not iceberg) lettuce, sliced tomatoes, a thin slice of reduced-fat cheddar, and gourmet mustard, and serve on a whole-grain bun.
- **Mashed Potatoes:** Substitute skim milk or fat-free half-and-half for whole milk, and cut the usual amount of butter in half. Throw in a few tablespoons of fat-free sour cream for a rich and creamy taste.
- **Sausage Pizza:** Top a ready-made pizza crust with tomato sauce; sliced bell peppers and red onions; pre-cooked and sliced chicken sausage links or crumbled turkey sausage; and a small amount of grated reduced-fat cheese.
- **Bacon and Eggs:** Scramble two egg whites and one whole egg. Serve with Canadian bacon, whole-wheat toast with marmalade, and fresh-squeezed orange juice.

and no one notices." You can shred carrots into spaghetti sauce, add vegetables to fajitas or burritos, and use oat bran in muffins. Puree vegetables, and add the liquid to cream sauces or soups; add spinach and crumbled tofu to lasagna; cook oatmeal in nonfat milk; mix wheat germ into your coating for chicken; use two egg whites instead of one whole egg in cooking. This way, you improve the entire family's diet and no one knows the difference.

Pump Up Flavor. To win over suspicious minds, make your healthy diet extra-yummy. "Even when other family members want to eat a healthier diet, you still need to make the foods taste great," says Donkersloot, who found that her husband would eat fruit if she brushed it with a little rum and grilled it lightly on the barbecue. That means using savory flavors, such as fresh herbs, garlic, chilies, ginger, lemon, sun-dried tomatoes, balsamic vinegar, horseradish, or salsa, for the adults in your house, while you might need to tone down flavors for little ones. Try mixing flavors, such as adding winter pears, fresh raspberries, or sliced peaches to a spinach salad. Skip the cutesy garnishes and the finely chopped celery, and focus on the type of meals most men like best—straightforward, uncomplicated, and satisfying.

Let 'em Splurge. Family members are much more likely to jump on board your healthy eating plan if they know they can still have their favorite junk food once in a while. "An occasional treat will go a long way in keeping your family on a healthy eating style," says Tribole. "When they feel deprived, they're likely to fight you tooth and nail." If having ice cream or soft drinks in the house leads to out-of-control bingeing, then don't stockpile these items and instead make the treat an excuse for an occasional family outing to the ice cream parlor or drive-through.

To create an eating plan that nurtures your health while satisfying your family's taste buds, you must develop meals that have something for everyone. Choose foods that do double duty—ones that are low in calories and fat but high in nutrients, fiber, and protective phytochemicals. Base your meals on real foods—such as vegetables, fruits, whole grains, legumes, and nuts—that will help you keep lean thighs as well as the strength and good health to power them. Then find an acceptable balance with your family's favorite items. For example, you might serve your children's favorite meal—hot dogs and baked beans—but accompany it with coleslaw made with low-fat dressing, orange segments, and nonfat milk. Mac and cheese out of the box still can be a quick-fix dinner; just prepare it with low-fat milk, and serve it with steamed broccoli and a quick salad. Hamburgers can be a regular favorite; just keep the servings small, and fill up on the green beans, sugar-free applesauce, and Caesar salad.

Granted, aiming to eat well for yourself might seem overwhelming when you're confronted with the demands and pressures of partners, children, and friends. Think positively. You can use your personal health goals for the betterment of your family. Many women report that as their diets improved, their husbands' blood pressure, cholesterol, and even waistlines, decreased. The sooner you start, the better, but it's never too late to introduce your children to healthful eating that will lower their risk for disease today and in the future. Besides, study after study has found that home-cooked meals are more nutritious than restaurant fare. So, you're already on the winning side of nutrition by just staying home!

Finally, on those nights when time constraints or the children's demands for takeout get the better of you, consider focusing on other meals. One woman gave in to her family's wishes at dinner but ate whole-grain cereal with light soy milk for breakfast and always took a healthy brown-bag lunch to work.

Serving Solutions

If your pressure problems come when you're dining out, keep in mind that you don't have to eat less or downsize portions—just eat better. "It's not bigger portions that cause weight problems," says Barbara Rolls, Ph.D., professor of nutrition at Pennsylvania State University. "It's bigger portions of foods high in fat, sugar, and calories." Help yourself to buckets of vegetables, broth-based soups, fruits, whole grains, and other real foods high in water and fiber, and you fill up before you fill out. For example, at a restaurant, select a chicken-and-vegetable soup and salad (dressing on the side) instead of an entree, ask if you can switch the baked potato for an extra serving of green beans to accompany your grilled salmon, or order oatmeal instead of an omelet.

Regardless of what's on the plate, it's up to you to take charge of how much you eat. Split an entree with a partner, request half orders, order à la carte, or bag half your entree before you begin to eat. You can order a high-calorie item, such as pasta Alfredo, but plan ahead by eating lightly during the day so that you budget enough calories to splurge.

Another solution is to order healthy items, such as a grilled-salmon spinach salad. A recent study found that eating your salad first fills you up, so you cut your portion of the main course and save yourself more than 100 calories! If you can't find just the right item, sweet-talk the staff into making substitutions or small changes in an entree, such as asking that the shish kebab be made with chicken breast instead of high-fat beef, or that the vegetables be steamed rather than sautéed in butter. At the drive-through, order a grilled chicken-breast sandwich with no mayo and a glass of orange juice, or split a burger and round out the meal with baby carrots and soy milk from home. Better yet, save high-calorie, fast-food meals for a once-a-month special occasion.

Keep Your Diet in Perspective

If the battle over what you should eat continues to rage either inside or outside your home, you might consider seeking help from a dietitian, counselor, or family physician. That partner, family member, or friend who won't listen to you may be willing to listen to someone else. Of course, if you want a direct answer to the question "How do I get my family to eat better, so I won't be tempted to overeat?" you have to ask them. In a straightforward, nonjudgmental way, explain that your concerns are about taking care of yourself and them.

Eating well should help you enjoy life more, not add additional stress. Nourishing your body with healthy food in healthy amounts should be a priority, not a punishment. Don't be too hard on yourself if you cave in to pressure or convenience once

My Plan to Fend Off Pressures to Eat

Think of a situation in which you are tempted by other people to overeat. This is what is called a "key situation" for you. It is an occasion when you are at high risk for veering from your best intentions to eat well. Your key situation will involve other people but also could include a particular place (a restaurant, a friend's house, a buffet), a particular time of day (a family member might be more likely to pressure you to eat at dinner than at breakfast), or even particular foods (your spouse tempts you by bringing home chocolate or chips). You need a plan, a strategy you develop ahead of time to fend off these pressures. Use this sheet to create your plan.

Situation	Important Factors (who, what, where, when)	Brainstorm Strategies
_____	_____	_____
_____	_____	_____
_____	_____	_____
_____	_____	_____
_____	_____	_____
_____	_____	_____
_____	_____	_____
_____	_____	_____

in a while. Juggling family, work, exercise, socializing, time demands, and all of life's responsibilities is anything but easy these days. Kim, a mother of three teenagers in Incline Village, Nevada, can attest to that. She confides, "I still have no clue how to maintain a balance in life while raising kids. I just decided not to beat myself up when I didn't do things perfectly. Instead, I focus on playing with my family, while trying to feed them a decent diet and keeping my sense of humor."

Not Being Honest

Stephanie, an elementary school teacher in San Diego, had a weight problem. Her cholesterol and blood sugar were on the rise, and given her family history of diabetes and heart disease, her physician had recommended that she lose at least 50 pounds. Now she was standing at my doorstep asking for diet advice.

On that first visit, I suggested she keep a food journal and write down everything she ate, how much, and when. A week later, the records showed that Stephanie already ate really well—lots of salads, few high-fat items, no soft drinks, and small portions. "I use lean cuts of meat, and I hardly ever snack," she emphasized. She agreed to make some adjustments in her eating style, such as including an additional vegetable at dinner, sautéing foods in chicken broth instead of olive oil, and eliminating the second piece of toast in the morning. Stephanie said she exercised regularly, but she promised to increase her workouts by 15 minutes at each session.

Weeks went by, and she lost only a few pounds. It didn't make sense. How could she eat so little and exercise so much, yet not drop more weight? She confirmed that this had been a problem for years: she didn't eat "anything," and certainly no more than any of her friends, yet the weight crept up, 5 to 10 pounds a year. Something was amiss.

That's when I decided to try a different tactic. I had Stephanie resume record keeping, but this time I asked her to use two different-colored pens. I told her to use a black pen to write down everything she ate and to use a red pen to write down everything she *would have eaten* if she hadn't been keeping records that I would review. I also reminded her how important it was to be completely honest and accurate in her record keeping. If that meant she weighed and measured her food for a full week, so be it.

The next week, Stephanie arrived at my office with a sheepish grin. This time the story was entirely different. She reported that during the week, she found herself writing in red ink more and more, which was an eye-opener. She now realized that she routinely ate more than she let on, much more. She told me, "Not mentioning certain snacks wasn't really intentional. I just didn't want to admit I was nibbling on the kids' old Halloween candy, and I justified the omission by telling myself that one little piece wouldn't make that big a difference." But it was one little piece over and over again throughout the day, plus a handful of chips and an extra serving of mashed potatoes. By weighing and measuring her food, Stephanie realized that what she'd considered a moderate portion was actually two to three times too big. All of this added up to several hundred excess calories every day.

Later in the session, Stephanie also conceded that she probably wasn't exercising as much as she'd said. She intended to go to the gym three times a week, but the weather had been bad, and more often than not, she made the drive only once or twice. She still exercised more than her friends, so in her mind, she had justified saying she worked out regularly. On my advice, Stephanie hired a personal trainer for a few sessions. The contrast between those sessions closely monitored by an expert and her previous workouts was another revelation. What Stephanie had thought was a vigorous workout wasn't even breaking a sweat, and her frequent stops at the water fountain and chats with gym mates meant that only about half of her 45-minute workout was actually spent moving. The end result: the calorie burn had been much lower than she had been estimating. "I never realized what a moderate workout was supposed to feel like until the personal trainer kept me moving constantly, and I mean constantly, for the hour," she said. "You could hardly call my past visits to the gym a workout in comparison!"

The good news is that once Stephanie was totally honest about what she was eating and how much she really was moving, the progress began. With some simple changes in her real food intake and her workout plans—rather than the imaginary diet and exercise program we had been working with—she lost the weight, and, more important, her blood cholesterol and sugar normalized, lowering her risk for disease down the road. Exercise also started to improve her life. She had more energy, better moods, less stress, and a feeling of real accomplishment, something that had eluded her when her activity level had been too low and sporadic.

Many women, like Stephanie, engage in battle against weight or health problems, yet their bodies seem resistant to change no matter which diet they go on and how hard they say they try. Sometimes these women have problems with fluid retention, in which fat loss is canceled out by the weight of the extra fluid. Luckily, fluid retention usually doesn't last, and within a few weeks of starting a healthy eating plan, the body flushes out the water, and the true loss shows on the scale. Other times, they have extremely low calorie requirements or sluggish metabolisms. These women must seriously amp up the activity level to jumpstart their metabolism or face a lifetime of existing on diets at near-fasting calorie levels. However, in most cases, this seeming defiance of the laws of physics—following a low-calorie diet and exercising vigorously, yet not dropping a pound—is simply a matter of not being completely honest about what's put on the plate and into the mouth, or how much, how vigorous, and how frequently the person exercises.

You are normal if you suspect you might be fudging portions or level of exercise. Inaccurate reporting is common; almost 8 out of every 10 of us do it to some degree. "Some people underreport everything they eat, even healthy food and how many vegetables they eat, but they really fudge on servings when it comes to desserts, snack items, and other foods high in fat and sugar," says Amy Subar, Ph.D., R.D., research nutritionist at the National Cancer Institute. On a happy note, once the whistle blows on dishonesty and women are given a few tools for accurately estimating how much they eat or how physically active they really are, their diets and exercise programs improve, they start dropping those unwanted pounds, and, like Stephanie, they feel better than they've felt in years.

Fessing Up Is Hard to Do

Ask most people what they ate yesterday, and odds are they will underestimate the intake. We all do it—lean or heavy, young or old, smokers or nonsmokers, athletes or couch potatoes. However, there is one consistent characteristic of underreporters: most of them are women—about two to one. One national nutrition survey found that women generally underestimate their daily food intake by approximately 800 calories! Even women who call themselves "small eaters" have been known to underreport their food intake by more than a third. In the case of Stephanie, who would have maintained a healthy weight on 2,200 calories a day, that one-third equated to more than 700 additional calories, for a day's total of 2,900 calories. The more overweight a woman is, or the more she overeats, the more she underestimates her food intake. The more fat and calories or potato chips, chocolate, ice cream, cakes, biscuits, alcohol, fatty cuts of meat, and other "naughty" foods she consumes, the more likely she is to fudge the numbers. The more a woman tends to diet, obsess over her weight, binge, or feel dissatisfied with her body image, the more likely she will lie—intentionally or unintentionally—about what she eats. In fact, overweight women eat up to twice as much as they report.

For some women, the dishonesty issue runs deep. One woman admitted that before she got honest about her food intake, it was not uncommon for her to squirrel food away in closets to eat when no one was looking. She ate an entire giant chocolate bunny after Easter and on several occasions made a batch of cookies, ate them all, and then baked a second batch so no one would know she had eaten the first. Yet, she never told anyone and continued to diet in public.

Those are the extremes. The rest of us mostly underreport the snacks we eat and downplay the fat in our diets. If we ate an entire batch of brownies while sitting at the computer, we'll say we had only a few or maybe not mention it at all. If we ate ice cream straight from the carton, we'll estimate that we had only a couple of bites, when in fact we downed a cup or more.

Sit-down meals are a different matter. While we are pretty honest about what we eat at meals, we also are likely to leave out certain details. So, we declare the generous serving of broccoli at dinner (a virtuous inclusion) but fail to mention that it was smothered in cheese sauce or dripping in butter. We admit we had some of our child's mac and cheese, but we swear the serving was minuscule, when in fact it was two heaping servings. As John Foreyt, Ph.D., director of the Behavioral Medicine Research Center at Baylor College of Medicine and an expert on weight management, sums up, "Women underreport having eaten foods at all, they forget to record how often they eat, and they really misrepresent their intake when it comes to portion sizes at a meal."

Do We Do It on Purpose?

We don't always mean to be dishonest about what we eat. "People often unintentionally misreport their food intake. They may have a hard time remembering what or how much they ate, or may feel pressured to report eating habits, so they unconsciously underreport," says Carmen D. Samuel-Hodge, Ph.D., of the University of North Carolina. There also is some downright confusion about what we should eat, and many of us don't have a clue about how much food is on our plates; we just serve it, eat it, and stop when we are full. Another reason could be that we're just caught up in the trend: more women underreport their food intake today than they did in the past.

Then again, others of us just plain lie. In one study, 68 percent of people admitted they were tempted to fib about their food intake during a dietary-recall questionnaire. "Who wants to admit to the unhealthy, fattening, or 'bad-for-you' foods?" one woman exclaimed. Instead, we are most likely to report what we should have eaten or what we think other people think we should eat, rather than what we actually ate. In a study from the University of North Carolina, 81 percent of women with diabetes said they ate less than they really did. They described their diets as matching the dietary guidelines for people with diabetes, when in truth their intakes were nowhere near that healthy.

Underscoring the irony, according to a study from the University of Hawaii, most of us know that the American diet is too high in calories and fat, and that portions are too big, but most of us also don't think that we are the ones who are eating too much. Instead, fewer than 20 percent of women rate their diets as high in fat, and only 10 percent rate their fat consumption as too high. This is in sharp contrast to a wealth of research that repeatedly and consistently shows just the opposite. These diet optimists are eating diets that increase their risks for all age-related diseases, including heart disease, diabetes, hypertension, and cancer, as well as memory loss. Because they describe their diets with a silver lining, they are oblivious to the fact that they need to drastically and immediately change their eating habits to sidestep disease down the road. (The Introduction has more details on women's eating habits.)

Exercise: Excuse Me!

While we downplay our doughnut indulgences, we play up our exercise. Like Stephanie, we often overestimate how often, how vigorously, and how long we work out. In a study from the University of Florida, 47 percent of exercisers said they worked out in moderation (the equivalent of a brisk walk), yet heart rate monitors told a different story. In fact, only 15 percent of those exercisers actually met this goal. While 11 percent reported that they exercised vigorously, such as jogging, only 2 percent actually did.

If you are spending more time at the gym, that's great. But don't make the mistake many women do of thinking that you exercise more than you do or that completing the four or five 30-minute workouts a week gives you carte blanche to eat whatever and whenever you want. The "I worked out today, so I can eat this" mentality can easily undermine your efforts at making healthful changes in your diet plan. In short, exercise is a critical part of a healthy lifestyle and weight-management plan, but it's not a justification of poor eating habits.

Some women who avoid exercise altogether justify their lack of activity by saying they lead active lives. Granted, if your active life is one in which you train horses, stack wood, or do heavy yard work all day, then you probably don't need to burn any more calories at the gym. However, it's rare for our modern-day lives to require that type of activity on a daily basis. More frequently, we think our lives are active because we chase kids, clean house, and run errands. That might enable you to maintain your weight when in your teens and twenties, but by the time most women hit their thirties, they must adopt structured exercise programs. If they don't, they begin to trade muscle for fat, gain weight as a result of sluggish metabolism, and get caught in the slow process that leads to disease and disability.

Any or all of these seemingly minor indiscretions when it comes to exercise can have big-time effects on our best efforts to lose weight and be healthier, both today and in the future. In essence, we become our own worst enemies, desperately wanting to be healthier, yet stabbing ourselves in the back by not being completely honest about what needs changing.

The Consequences of Not Being Honest

Don't get me wrong: optimism is certainly an admirable quality in many aspects of life. Believing you can succeed, for example, is a powerful attitude for making any change. But when optimism is used as a form of diet or exercise denial, it can get in your way of any real and permanent change for the better. If you think you're doing pretty well, eating right and exercising enough, you have no reason to change or improve. Fibbing makes it impossible to identify what you're doing wrong so that it can be fixed. As a consequence, you forfeit your right to control your health and well-being. In effect, you're saying, "I am powerless to be better. I've tried, and nothing works." This attitude undermines your hopes, self-esteem, motivation, and confidence. The truth is you can change; you can lose weight; you can be healthier, more energetic, mentally sharper, and able to enjoy life to its fullest. That change comes from within, and it starts with honestly scrutinizing your diet and activity habits.

Just becoming aware that you haven't been completely accurate or honest in your diet reporting is enough to begin the journey toward success. Numerous studies show that women's reporting improves substantially with some gentle reminders to be totally honest about food servings and activity levels. They also get healthier and leaner. In fact, dietitians and other nutrition experts have found that sometimes all it takes for their clients to achieve weight-loss goals is to ask them to write down their food and exercise habits.

Portion Distortion

A key area of nutrition on which to focus is people's distorted perspective of what constitutes a portion. While you're cutting back on pasta and bread, adding more meat or tuna, or switching to fat-free items at the grocery store, you could be missing the point: the problem when it comes to getting real about your dietary habits could be how much, not what, you're eating. "People are so focused on fat or carbs that they are blind to the huge portions of energy-dense foods they are being served," says Barbara Rolls, Ph.D., of Pennsylvania State University, author of *The Volumetrics Weight-Control Plan: Feel Full on Fewer Calories*. As a result, we are gobbling 15 percent more calories today than we did 20 years ago.

Portions have ballooned as much as eightfold in the past 30 years, both inside and outside the home, with the greatest increases coming in calorie-packed fast food, such as refined grains, meat, and soft drinks. Lisa Young, Ph.D., of New York University, researched portions and found that, compared with 20 years ago, a typical bakery cookie today is eight times larger, a serving of pasta is almost six times larger, coffee-shop muffins and bagels are three times larger, and a typical serving of restaurant steak is twice as large. "Restaurants are using larger plates, bakers are using bigger muffin tins, pizzerias are using larger pans,

Can You Tell a Muffin from a Cake?

Test your portion distortion by taking this quiz. These standard servings are established by the U.S. Department of Agriculture (USDA) and are used for making dietary recommendations, including those in the Food Guide Pyramid.

Vegetables and Fruits
1. A serving of raw fruits or vegetables is 1 cup, which is the size of:
   a. a Ping Pong ball
   b. a baseball
   c. a racquetball
   d. a basketball
2. A serving of cooked fruits or vegetables is ½ cup, which is the size of:
   a. an ice cream scoop
   b. a small container of yogurt
   c. a yo-yo
   d. a soup bowl

Grains (preferably whole grains)
3. A 2-ounce bagel or muffin is a serving of grain and is about the size of:
   a. a tennis ball
   b. a Ping Pong ball
   c. a soccer ball
   d. a marble
4. A serving of cooked brown rice, oatmeal, polenta, or pasta is ½ cup and is about the size of:
   a. a cupped hand
   b. two cupped hands
   c. a tennis ball
   d. a Frisbee

continued

Milk Products or Soy Milk

5. A serving of nonfat milk, soy milk, or yogurt is 1 cup and is about the size of:
   a. a water bottle
   b. a wineglass
   c. a baseball
   d. a can of soda pop
6. A serving of cheese is 1½ ounces, which is the size of:
   a. a tight fist
   b. a CD case
   c. four marshmallows
   d. a 9-volt battery

Meat and Beans

7. A serving of meat is 3 ounces, or the size of:
   a. a deck of cards
   b. a compact CD player
   c. a hockey puck
   d. a romance novel
8. A serving of peanut butter is 2 tablespoons, which is the size of:
   a. a tangerine
   b. a TV remote control
   c. a marble
   d. an Oreo cookie
9. A serving of black beans is ½ cup, which is the size of:
   a. a daisy
   b. a sunflower
   c. a rose
   d. a large tulip

Fats (no more than 30 percent of total calories)

10. For fat, such as butter, oil, margarine, or shortening, 1 teaspoon is equivalent to:
    a. a postage stamp
    b. a lipstick tube

c. a thumb
d. a Ping Pong ball

Answers: 1. b; 2. a; 3. b; 4. c; 5. c ; 6. d ; 7. a; 8. d; 9. d;
10. a

Your score:

9–10: Excellent! You're a portion guru, well versed in how
to spot too much of what.

6–8: Good. You're right more often than not, but be careful of unwanted calories sneaking into your diet from too-
big portions.

4–5: Poor. Back to school, girl, to learn what's a portion
and what's a platter.

< 4: Horrible. Quick, buy a food scale and a measuring cup,
and get to work before you break any more portion rules.

cars have larger cup holders, and fast-food restaurants are pack-
aging drinks and french fries in bigger containers," says Young.
The upshot is that we eat more without realizing it.

There are the obvious culprits, such as 7-Eleven's 64-ounce
Big Gulp, which packs almost 800 calories and requires two
hands to lift. Then there are the sneaky ones, such as McDonald's hamburgers, which have gradually mushroomed from their
original 3.9 ounces and 280 calories (about the size of a kid's
Happy Meal burger by today's standards) to the Double Quarter
Pounder with Cheese at 9.9 ounces, 770 calories, and 70 percent
of your total day's allotment for fat. Even the small buckets of
popcorn, bags of candy and chips, cans of pop, and you name it
are best shared by two or more people, if eaten at all. It's no wonder people have totally lost track of what a real portion should
look like!

Portion Shockers

- A Cinnabon's Caramel Pecanbon weighs half a pound and packs in 900 calories, more than 10 teaspoons of fat, and two-thirds of the day's allotment for saturated fat, which makes the original Cinnabon look almost like diet food at only 670 calories, 8½ teaspoons of fat, and 14 grams of saturated fat!
- A Crispy Chicken Caesar Salad at McDonald's with croutons and a packet of dressing supplies 550 calories, the calorie equivalent of a Quarter Pounder with Cheese and half of your day's allotment of fat (35.5 grams, or 9 teaspoons).
- An Au Bon Pain Chocolate Chip Muffin weighs 4.5 ounces and supplies 600 calories, 26 grams of fat, and 6 grams of saturated fat.
- A Starbucks Blueberry Crumb Cake weighs 7 ounces and contains 800 calories, 9½ teaspoons of fat, and 18 grams of saturated fat.
- A Baja Fresh Dos Manos Enchilada Style Burrito weighs 62 ounces and contains 3,370 calories, 39 teaspoons of fat, and 63 grams of saturated fat.
- A Rubio's Baja Grill Combo packs in 1,460 calories, 66 grams of fat, and 17 grams of saturated fat.
- A Baskin-Robbins Vanilla Shake (large) weighs a pound and a half and supplies 1,070 calories and 32 saturated fat grams.
- TCBY's Toffee Coffee Cappuccino Chiller (large) has 1,200 calories and 30 grams of saturated fat.
- A Nestle Toll House Cookie Ice Cream Sandwich packs in 540 calories, along with 6½ teaspoons of fat, of which 11 grams are saturated fat.
- A Starbucks Café Mocha Grande made with whole milk contains 409 calories and almost 8 teaspoons of fat, which is the calorie equivalent of eating one and a half pieces of devil's food cake with frosting, but with twice the fat.

As we grow accustomed to gigantic servings, our portion awareness gets thrown totally out of whack. One study found that when asked to eyeball what they considered a "medium" serving, people estimated it as much bigger than standard serving sizes. Here are a few examples of people's reported distortions:

- A typical "medium" serving of meat—8 ounces, not the 3 ounces established by the USDA
- A typical "medium" muffin—6 ounces, three times the USDA's 2 ounces
- A typical "medium" baked potato—7 ounces, versus the USDA's 4 ounces

Forks Versus Forklifts

A subtle way in which people are enticed to eat more is with bigger containers of food. "People eat in units, such as a sandwich, a cookie, a plate of food, a bag of chips, a slice of pizza. Today these units are jumbo burgers, bigger plates, and muffins the size of small cakes," says Paul Rozin, M.D., of the University of Pennsylvania, who has compared portions in the United States and France. With almost 7 out of every 10 of us "cleaning our plates," the calories quickly add up.

Brian Wansink, Ph.D., professor of consumer psychology at the University of Illinois, Urbana-Champaign, has investigated what cues people to eat more and found that people eat more when served more. In one study, people ate 39 percent more M&Ms candies when munching from a big bag than they did when given small bags. And with a 50 percent increase in snacking over the past 20 years, that's a lot of extra calories. In study after study, people eat up to 45 percent more food when served bigger helpings. In a study from Pennsylvania State University, when people were offered four different portions of the same lunch over a span of several weeks, they ate 30 percent more calories when offered the largest portion, yet half of the eaters didn't notice a difference in the serving size. "Our feeling of fullness adjusts to the amount of food in front of us. Give bigger portions, and people take bigger bites and eat more, yet end up with the

What's a Portion?

Following are the number of recommended servings per day for each food group, according to the USDA, and some sample servings.

- Fruits and Vegetables: 8 to 10+ servings per day
  - Raw: 1 cup or 1 medium piece
  - Cooked/canned: ½ cup
- Grains (preferably whole grains): 6+ servings per day
  - 1 slice of bread
  - ½ cup of cooked pasta, rice, or hot cereal
  - Half of a hamburger bun
  - 1 3-ounce bagel or English muffin
- Milk products: 3 servings per day
  - 1 cup of milk or yogurt
  - 1 ounce of cheese
  - ½ cup of cottage cheese
- Legumes/Meat: 2–3 servings per day
  - 3 ounces of meat, chicken, or fish, cooked
  - ½ cup of cooked dried beans or peas
- Nuts/Seeds: 1 ounce per day
- Fats: 1 teaspoon of butter, margarine, or oil

same feelings of fullness, all of which leads to greater food intake," says Barbara Rolls, head researcher on the study.

Just the sight of food can entice us to eat. Wansink placed chocolate kisses in glass or opaque bowls either on people's desks or six feet away. On average, "People ate only four chocolates when they had to get up for a treat, six if the chocolates were close at hand but in opaque bowls, and nine chocolates when they were in a clear bowl on the desk," says Wansink. "How food is served determines the portion, too. Put soda pop in a short, fat glass, and people drink more and think they are drinking less than when it's in a tall, thin glass. So, the shape of the glass can make a difference," says Wansink. He warns, "In our land of plenty, the last thing women should do to curb portions is rely on willpower and diligence. Left to these faulty devices, most people will eat and drink too much."

Kick the Habit

The most important tool for getting a handle on your true eating and exercise habits is to keep a journal. As mentioned in Habit 1: Mindless Eating, record keeping is the number one trait shared by people who successfully change their eating habits for good and maintain their weight loss. Review the nuts and bolts of record keeping from Habit 1, and vow to keep a journal for at least a week. As I advised Stephanie, use two different-colored pens, one to write down what you eat and the other to write down what you would have eaten if you weren't obliged to admit it on paper. Be honest and accurate about everything you eat and drink. "Just the act of recording your food intake often is enough to help you tone down the unwanted calories or bad habits," says Susan Moores, M.S., R.D., spokesperson for the American Dietetic Association.

Remember that food records are only as useful as the accuracy of the information in them. If you keep records, make a few changes, and still don't lose weight, you may need to do some record-keeping adjustments. "People typically underestimate their overall food intake by about a third, so for people to be truly honest about their calorie balance, I recommend that they keep food journals and then add at least a third more calories to their reported daily total," says Baylor's John Foreyt. Of course, knowing how much you should be eating and getting a handle on those portions is a must, too.

Weigh and Measure Your Food

Portion vigilance could be the only tool you need to nudge your diet and your waistline into line. It is a critical component when keeping food records. Miscalculate your portions, especially for

How Much Should You Be Eating?

Record keeping helps you figure out what you're eating, but how does that compare with what you should be eating? What does a 1,200-calorie diet look like? A 1,500-calorie diet? Or a 2,000-calorie diet? The calories pile up more easily than you might think. Here are examples to help guide your choices.

A 1,200-Calorie Diet

Breakfast: A 1-ounce serving of cereal with 1 cup of non-fat milk and a piece of fruit

Lunch: A turkey sandwich on whole-wheat bread with mustard, 2 cups of tossed salad with 1 tablespoon of fat-free dressing, and a 6-ounce container of yogurt

Dinner: 3 ounces of lean meat or chicken, a small sweet potato, and ½ cup of cooked rice

Snacks: An orange

A 1,500-Calorie Diet

Breakfast: A 1-ounce serving of cereal with 1 cup of non-fat milk and a piece of fruit

Lunch: A turkey sandwich on whole-wheat bread with mustard, 2 cups of tossed salad with 1 tablespoon of fat-free dressing, and a 6-ounce container of yogurt

Dinner: 3 ounces of lean meat or chicken, a small sweet potato, 1 cup of steamed broccoli, and ½ cup of cooked rice

Snacks: An orange, a glass of nonfat milk, and 1 cup of strawberries dunked in ¼ cup of chocolate syrup

A 2,000-Calorie Diet

Breakfast: A 2-ounce serving of cereal with 1 cup of non-fat milk, topped with walnuts and 1 tablespoon of Craisins, and a piece of fruit

Lunch: A turkey sandwich on whole-wheat bread with mustard, 3 cups of tossed salad with 2 tablespoons of regular ranch dressing, and a 6-ounce container of yogurt

Dinner: 3 ounces of lean meat or chicken, a small sweet potato, 1 cup of steamed broccoli, and 1 cup of cooked rice

Snacks: An orange, a glass of nonfat milk, and 1 cup of strawberries dunked in ¼ cup of chocolate syrup

high-fat or high-sugar items, and your records become next to useless for gauging your calorie and nutrient intake.

"People take their cues about what constitutes a serving by what they see in restaurants, where too much food is heaped onto too-big plates," says Lisa Young. The solution here is to measure and weigh your food at home for a week to hone your portion-awareness skills (using the listings under "What's a Portion?" earlier in this chapter as a guide). You'll need a food scale and a set of measuring cups. Make a vow for one week to serve yourself your customary portions, and weigh or measure them to see how closely they fit the ideal. Pare down any portions that exceed the recommended servings. Your goal is to stick closely to the serving sizes for grains, fats, oils, cheese, nuts, and meat and to be generous with your helpings of salad, fruit, and vegetables. For example, you may find when you measure your plate of pasta that you have served yourself 4 cups, the equivalent of eight USDA standard servings of grain—more than a day's worth. Or, that "generous" serving of broccoli may be only ½ cup, which is not generous, just standard. The 2 tablespoons of green peas in your soup or the tablespoon of blueberries in a muffin do not a portion make, but the scone you had with your coffee actually weighed in at 5 ounces, not the 1½ ounces suggested by the USDA as a serving.

Yes, weighing and measuring is time-consuming. Yes, it is a hassle. But it's necessary, and you'll need to do it for only a week to get real about how much you're eating and to learn how to eyeball accurate portions of your favorite foods. As Paul Rozin says, "You must engineer your world to reduce portions." Weighing and measuring is a great place to start. It's also a good habit to return to when the pounds start creeping back on. Here are two more ways to help ensure that your portions are accurate:

- Ask your butcher to cut meat and fish into 4-ounce portions.
- Weigh portions at the store, such as russet potatoes (purchase 8-ouncers and cut them in half at home).

Scale Down Packaged and Fast Foods

There are a few additional habits to adopt. Watch out for the "more is better" mentality, especially with snack foods and fast foods. Advertisements and fast-food menus entice us to buy larger-size portions, implying a better value for our money. True, a supersized value meal or an economy-size bag of chips might be good for your wallet, but it wreaks havoc with your waistline and health. Labels can be misleading, giving us the impression we're eating less than we are. The number of calories might be listed as 150, but if there are three servings in the bag and you eat it all, you've tripled your calorie intake to 450 calories!

Packaged foods almost always are too big. "You must construct an environment that makes it difficult to overeat big portions of highly processed snack foods," suggests Wansink. That means adopting a portion-savvy attitude:

- Divvy up packages into smaller portions.
- Share anything that comes in an individual wrapper.
- Store foods away from sight, such as in the basement, since the very sight of food can lead us to eat.
- On the other hand, use the sight of food to your advantage by placing pictures of salad and vegetables in clear view, a bowl of blueberries on your desk for an afternoon snack, and cut-up fresh fruit on the table after dinner.
- Skip the "value" meals and "economy-size" bags of munchies.
- Serve meals on salad plates and in small bowls.
- Share a small bag of candy at the theater. (Better yet, take along your own healthy snacks from home!)
- Leave food on your plate.
- Order a kid's hamburger instead of the Big Mac.

At restaurants, in airplanes, at buffet tables, and at social gatherings, really take a look at what ends up on your plate. "Just because the food is put in front of you doesn't mean you have to eat it all," says Young.

Diet 101

If lack of knowledge is the reason you are less than accurate about what you eat, then the answer is easy—boost your nutrition know-how.

Get Fat-Free and Low-Carb Savvy. "What a fat-free cookie loses in fat it gains in sugar, and what a low-carb snack bar loses in sugar it gains in fat; consequently, most of these processed desserts have about the same calories as regular ones," warns Adam Drewnowski, Ph.D., professor in the Departments of Epidemiology and Medicine at the University of Washington. Fat-free cream cheese may be lower in calories, but not if you slather three times as much on a bagel. Use sparingly both regular and fat-free versions of anything sweet or creamy, and venture into the low-carb arena with a very wary eye.

Read Labels. Look for foods that supply no more than 3 grams of fat for every 100 calories. Also, note the printed serving size, which might be unrealistically small, giving the false impression that the food is low-calorie.

Never Socialize on an Empty Stomach. People eat more when they're with friends and family. Have a healthful snack before a party, split an entree when dining out, and don't mix alcohol with socializing, since even one drink can derail the best of intentions, leaving you more likely to overeat. (See Habit 9: Drinking Away Our Waistlines for more information on how alcohol interferes with weight and health management.)

Do the Grease Slick Test. Some foods don't come with labels, such as that bran muffin at the coffee shop or the doughnuts after church. Still, you usually can tell that something is high in fat by the slick feel in your mouth. Likewise, if your doughnut leaves your fingers or napkin greasy, you can bet several teaspoons of fat went into its making.

Take Conscious Control. "Make a conscious decision to choose more fruits, vegetables, and whole grains, and you automatically will reduce the calories, fat, and sugar in your diet," asserts Drewnowski.

How Much Exercise Is Enough?

Choosing a couch-potato lifestyle is no laughing matter. "If you are sedentary, you have the same risk of dying prematurely as a person who smokes a pack a day," says Kenneth Cooper, M.D., M.P.H., founder of the Cooper Institute of Aerobics Research, in Dallas. A sedentary lifestyle is even more of a health threat than high blood pressure, obesity, family history of disease, or high cholesterol. No doubt about it: whatever your health or weight goals, you must exercise. The question is, how much?

Your minimum goal is to burn 150 calories or more a day, or about 1,000 calories a week. That's about half an hour every day, seven days a week, of moderate activity, defined as any activity that boosts your heart rate to the level of brisk walking. You can exercise continually for 30 minutes, or break up this activity into minisessions—such as three 10-minute stair-climbing sessions or two 15-minute stints on the exercise bicycle. To build and maintain muscle—which you begin to lose by your thirties—you also should plan two strength-training sessions a week. That is the minimum. The more you do and the more vigorous the workout, the greater the benefits to your health. However, anyone who has a chronic disease or who is over 40 years old should consult a physician before beginning an activity program.

For weight loss, you'll need to amp up the exercise quotient even more. "No diet on the planet will maintain a healthy weight if you don't exercise," says Jim Hill, Ph.D., cofounder of the National Weight Control Registry (NWCR) and author of *The Step Diet: Count Steps, Not Calories, to Lose Weight and Keep It Off Forever*. People who successfully lose weight and maintain the loss move much more than the half hour a day recommended for general health. "They get lots of exercise—the equivalent of an hour or more a day, or 28 miles of brisk walking a week—which means they probably have much less time to veg out in front of the TV," says Suzanne Phelan, Ph.D., coinvestigator in the NWCR and assistant professor of psychology at Brown University. "The more weight you want to lose, and the more you need to maintain that loss, the more you have to move," adds Hill.

Researchers don't understand why a formerly obese person must exercise more than an always-lean person to maintain the lower weight, although Hill speculates that it probably relates to some kind of permanent metabolic slowdown that results from having been obese. "It's not fair that you need to move 12,000 steps a day, while your skinny neighbor might need only 8,000 steps, but that's the reality," he concludes. To spice up their active lives, diet masters turn to variety, with 6 out of every 10 masters incorporating two or more types of exercise into their weekly routines.

Steppin' Out

Someone who wants to lose 30 or more pounds and maintain the loss will need to increase her daily movement *and* exercise a lot. First, start defining yourself as someone who is active. Then, follow Hill's advice to purchase a pedometer (one comes with his book) and plan to take 8,000 steps during the day, by using stairs instead of the elevator, getting up to change the TV channel instead of clicking the remote, and walking to the neighbor's house instead of calling. In addition, exercise almost every day. People in the NWCR, an ongoing study of people who have lost a significant amount of weight and maintained the loss, burn about 400 calories a day in exercise alone, the equivalent of about one hour, or walking four miles.

While this might sound daunting to the novice, keep in mind that some exercise is better than none, and even a slight boost in activity can bring emotional and health benefits. Also, give yourself time to reach your exercise goals. "Masters didn't start out exercising for an hour every day; they worked up to that level over time," says Hill. This means some serious soul-searching about your goals for weight and health management.

Goal Setting

This chapter is all about being honest, gathering accurate information about what you eat and how much you exercise. That information is useful and essential to meeting your goals to be healthier or lose a few pounds. What you do with your new information will depend on where you want to go with your health.

Goals are your road map to managing your diet and your weight. Without goals, you won't know where you are going or even if you got there. For a goal to be useful, it must be specific, realistic, and flexible.

Specific Goals Are Measurable. Instead of a vague goal to "exercise more" or "reduce fat intake," write specific goals that include *what*, *when*, *where*, and *how*, such as, "I will jog for 30 minutes during my lunch hour, five days a week, for the next six months," or "To reduce my fat intake, I will spread apple butter instead of butter on my toast in the morning."

Get Real. Realistic goals take into account where you are today and what you are likely to accomplish with reasonable effort. Unrealistic goals are a setup for failure, so avoid perfectionist goals that use words such as *always*, *never*, or *every day*. (One way to test a goal is to ask yourself, "Would I expect a friend to meet these expectations?") For a goal to be realistic, it should be broken down into ministeps.

The path to long-term success is lined with hundreds of small accomplishments. For example, a long-term goal to lose 20 pounds can be broken down into short-term goals to lose 1 to 2 pounds a week for the next 10 to 20 weeks. The ministeps you use to reach that short-term goal can be outlined on the work sheet, "My Road Map to Success," at the end of this chapter and might include walking an additional three miles a day to burn 250 calories, replacing negative thoughts with supportive thoughts, and substituting baby carrots for potato chips at the midafternoon snack.

Stay Flexible. Modify your ministeps if you find they are either too easy or too difficult. Goals should be challenging, not overwhelming.

Finally, strive for goals that you personally want, not goals someone else says you should attain.

It's Within Your Grasp

It is not easy being honest about sensitive issues, such as weight or eating and exercise habits. It is no fun to admit you have been less than perfect, perhaps even downright lazy. It is hard medicine to swallow when you must admit that you are responsible for where your health and weight is today; you can't blame it on

My Road Map to Success

Complete the following work sheet each week. (Use this sheet as a master copy.) After you've listed your ministep goals for the week, use the checklist to monitor your success: Give yourself credit by making a tally mark under the appropriate day each time you accomplish a ministep. There can be more than one tally mark per day.

Date/Week: _____

Long-Term Goal: _____

This Week's Short-Term Goal: _____

Ministep Goals (include details such as when, where, how often, with whom):

1. _____

2. _____

3. _____

	Mon.	Tue.	Wed.	Thu.	Fri.	Sat.	Sun.
Ministep 1	__	__	__	__	__	__	__
Ministep 2	__	__	__	__	__	__	__
Ministep 3	__	__	__	__	__	__	__

an underactive gland, a sluggish metabolism, or a lifestyle too busy for exercise. On a positive note, because you are the only one who can change you, the power to make those changes—to be the healthiest, the fittest, the happiest, the best person you can be—is completely within your grasp. The steps are easy: For one week, weigh and measure your food, time your exercise, and write it all down. Review your records, set your goals, and then start tweaking those aspects of your life that are confounding your efforts to feel and look great.

Skip the Broccoli, Eat the Fries

If you were to do nothing else but double your current intake of fruits and vegetables, you'd be well on your way to eating a good diet. I've seen it happen over and over, but probably nowhere was this one tip more useful than when I worked with Sue, a graphic artist from the Boston area, as part of a series called "New Year, New You" for ABC's "Good Morning America." Sue wanted to lose the postpregnancy 20 pounds and drop a clothing size. The advice was simple, the time investment was nil, and she exceeded her wildest dreams, dropping three clothing sizes! "When people ask me how I did it, I have to stop and think. Losing weight had always been such a monumental task in the past, but this time it took so little effort or time that I hardly even knew I was dieting," says Sue.

Sue's eating habits were pretty typical. She was skipping meals, grabbing fatty convenience foods on the run, and not eating enough fruits and vegetables. So it goes for most women. According to the U.S. Department of Agriculture's Continuing Survey of Food Intakes by Individuals, a measly 1 out of every 100 of us meets even minimum standards for dietary adequacy. One in every four of us doesn't include even one fruit in our daily diet, we average only three vegetables, and according to Gladys Block, Ph.D., professor of public health nutrition at the University of California,

Berkeley, as few as 7 percent of women consume even one dark green leafy vegetable on any four days (we need at least two daily).

Don't blame a time crunch for these poor diets. Sue lost weight with simple changes, ones that took little or no extra time. "Heaping half the plate with fruits and vegetables and not allowing anything in the house that had more than 3 grams of fat for every 100 calories were the two biggest time-savers," says Sue. In study after study, results affirm that people who eat the most fruits and vegetables are also the most likely to lose weight and maintain the weight loss. In a study from Northwestern University, in Chicago, women who ate the most fruits and vegetables had a 24 percent lower risk of obesity than those who ate little produce.

The benefits go far beyond just weight loss. Nothing wields a more powerful health punch than produce. From a crunchy apple, a juicy orange, or a sweet plum to a crisp spinach salad, a ripe tomato, or a creamy yam, all fruits and vegetables are good for us. "Thousands of studies spanning decades of research consistently and repeatedly show that women who eat diets rich in vegetables and fruit significantly lower their risks for most age-related diseases, from heart disease and diabetes to hypertension, cancer, and cataracts," says Jeffrey Blumberg, Ph.D., professor in the Friedman School of Nutrition Science and Policy at Tufts University.

A study from the Centers for Disease Control and Prevention concluded that not eating enough fruits and vegetables ranks second only to not using sunscreen as the most common significant health behavior contributing to disease risks. So, even if you don't focus on fat, even if you don't cut carbs or limit sweets, even if you don't give up your daily soft drink (of course, those changes are good, too!) but you do simply change your current eating habits to double your intake of produce—and you make those extra choices colorful ones—you will have taken the single greatest step toward a healthful diet and will dramatically improve your chances of side-stepping all age-related diseases that may lurk in the future.

Nothing Is Better for You than Produce

Heart disease is the leading cause of disability and death among women, and keeping your ticker healthy begins with fruits and vegetables. A study from the University of Toronto found that plant-based diets rich in fruits and vegetables were as effective as the leading statin medications for lowering cholesterol and the risk for heart disease. Produce raises the good cholesterol (HDLs), lowers both total and LDL cholesterol (the bad guys), and even reduces another marker of heart disease called homocysteine. The more fruits and vegetables you eat, the lower your risk, with women who eat 10 or more servings a day experiencing up to a 55 percent lower risk for heart disease compared with women who eat fewer than 3 a day.

A perfect example of the benefits of produce is the case with vegetarians, who might go through life tortured by the smell of barbecued ribs and frying bacon but who, in the long run, are healthier than their meat-eating friends. Several studies show that America's 15 million vegetarians have much lower rates of cancer and hypertension, and up to a 50 percent lower risk for heart disease, compared with the general public. They also have an easier time managing their weights, and they live longer. In fairness to meat, the real issue might not be the harmful effects of a T-bone steak, but rather the protective effects of the abundance of fruits and vegetables in the typical vegetarian diet.

If that weren't enough, produce also is one of the best defenses against cancer. Researchers estimate that at least 35 percent of cancer deaths could be avoided by diet alone, with fruits and vegetables leading the pack in cancer prevention. For example:

- Produce rich in vitamin C, such as oranges, red bell peppers, and grapefruit, lowers instances of cancers of the esophagus, stomach, lungs, cervix, colon, and pancreas.
- Carotene-rich mangoes, carrots, sweet potatoes, and papayas lower lung and liver cancer risk.
- Cruciferous vegetables, such as broccoli and cabbage, lower overall cancer risk.

That's just the tip of the iceberg. Heaping the plate with produce helps sidestep stroke, reduces symptoms of non-Hodgkin's lymphoma, builds bones that are resistant to osteoporosis, prevents urinary-tract infections, lowers the risk for diabetes and high blood pressure, and boosts the immune system. A produce-packed diet also helps prevent wrinkling and premature aging of the skin, so you look younger. You also feel and act younger, and live longer. According to a study from the University of Naples, in Italy, people who live more than a century also live the healthiest. Their secret? You guessed it: they eat the most fruits and vegetables.

Last but not least, as Sue found, generous servings of fruits and vegetables are a must for lifelong weight control. Women who battle weight problems inevitably consume too much high-calorie food and too few fruits and vegetables, while a study from Tufts University found that women who ate healthy diets rich in fruits and vegetables had the greatest success at weight management. Walter Willett, M.D., Dr.P.H., professor at the Harvard School of Public Health, sums it up by saying, "A main contributor to the diet-health issue is what we've done to our food supply. We've taken wholesome, nutritious foods such as corn and made partially hydrogenated corn oil and high-fructose corn syrup; then we throw away most of the good stuff. People would be much better off if they planned meals and snacks around minimally processed, real foods, such as fruits and vegetables."

Why Is Produce So Good for Us?

Most women know they should be eating more steamed broccoli and spinach salads. We know these are Mother Nature's perfect foods and the best dietary sources of antioxidants, such as vitamin C and beta-carotene. Antioxidants block highly reactive oxygen fragments called free radicals that otherwise damage the genetic code, cell membranes, and proteins, leading to aging, heart disease, cancer, and all the other diseases that antioxidants protect against. Produce also is a major contributor of fiber, which lowers your risk for heart disease, diabetes, and breast cancer and helps satisfy you on few calories.

What you may not know is that even if you take supplements and eat bran cereal, you can't make up for a lack of produce, since fruits and vegetables contain thousands of phytochemicals that boost defenses against most diseases—from d-limonene in citrus, ellagic acid in apples, and flavonoids in grapes to indoles in cauliflower, lycopene in tomatoes, and sulforaphane in broccoli. Most of these phytochemicals are antioxidants. For example, phytochemicals called polyphenols in grapes lower the risk for heart disease and stroke by preventing blood clots. Monoterpenes in oranges reduce cancer risk by triggering enzymes that break down cancer-causing substances. In latter stages of cancer, monoterpenes cause cancer cells to commit suicide, a type of cell death called apoptosis. Lycopene in tomatoes is a potent antioxidant that mops up free radicals associated with cancer and heart disease.

Many phytochemicals are in the pigments of fruits or vegetables. The intense reds and blues in berries come from anthocyanins, potent antioxidants that absorb free radicals. The red or yellow-orange hues in mangoes and carrots come from more than six hundred different antioxidants called carotenoids, of which beta-carotene, lycopene, and lutein are best known. The deeper the color, the higher the level of antioxidants. That means spinach is a better salad green than romaine lettuce, which in turn is much better than head lettuce, such as iceberg.

How Much Are You Eating?

How many vegetables and fruits do you routinely include in your daily diet? Be honest—don't exaggerate. If you're like most other women, you probably only give lip service to produce. We include three, maybe four, servings of something vegetable- or fruitlike on our daily plates, but we say we eat more than that number. Every national nutrition survey dating back to the late 1960s reports that Americans avoid fruit like the plague. Back in 1991, the National Cancer Institute established its "5-a-Day for Better Health" program to encourage Americans to eat more fruits and vegetables. (Not that there is anything magical about five servings. It's just that we're eating so few fruits and vegetables that boosting intake to even a measly five servings seemed like a manageable first-step goal.) Only 1 in every 10 of us meets this goal. Three out of every four fail to include three servings of fruit in their daily diets; half of us consume less than one serving. Despite all the scientific hullabaloo about eating more produce, our average daily consumption has inched up only 0.3 serving since the 1970s, the equivalent of an extra bite of broccoli.

Maybe it's because we didn't grow up eating produce-based diets. For example, Nancy, a magazine editor in Los Angeles, admits, "I grew up eating astronaut food. Swanson's TV dinners. Hostess Ding Dongs. Oscar Mayer bologna and Wonder Bread sandwiches. And, yes, Tang. Vegetables were something that came out of a Birds Eye bag, usually the peas-and-carrots mix. My siblings and I considered eating the desiccated vegetables to be a form of torture. Luckily, they appeared on the table only about once a week." Many other women I interviewed also commented that, for them, fruit was not a standard part of childhood. "Except for an occasional banana, my mother didn't like fruit, so it wasn't in our house. I was in college before I realized that the funny orange stuff on the hot-lunch buffet back in high school that I had thought might be Spam was actually *cantaloupe*," says Gretchen, a medical sales representative in Madison, Wisconsin.

Here are some other reasons proffered for why we skimp on vegetables, along with the counterarguments:

- **Produce is pricey.** "Fresh produce is expensive, so many people turn to cheaper foods that provide more calories per dollar, like fast food," says Adam Drewnowski, Ph.D., professor in the Departments of Epidemiology and Medicine at the University of Washington. Sure, price might play a part, but it can't be the determining factor. A study (mentioned at the beginning of this chapter) from the University of California, Berkeley, found that only 14 percent of women with money to burn included even one green leafy on any four days. Moreover, according to the U.S. Department of Agriculture (USDA), Americans are spending a smaller percentage of their dollars on food than ever before. We obviously aren't putting our money where our mouths are!

- **Produce is scarce.** Wait a minute. . . . Availability can't be the main issue, since produce variety has increased since the 1970s from 150 to more than 400 different selections. And produce departments have never been so big!
- **No time.** Hey, with so many quick-fix options available today, such as bagged lettuce and precut vegetables, this excuse appears a bit lame.

More likely, a major reason why we fail at produce consumption is that we don't realize how little we're eating. In studies from the University of Maastricht, in Netherlands, 88 percent of people who didn't include ample produce in their diets thought they were getting enough. Feeling the need to make a change is the number one motivator for cleaning up your diet, but people aren't likely to eat more broccoli if they think they're already doing just fine.

The Choices We Make

When we nibble on fruits and vegetables, the choices we make are often nutritional duds. Out of more than 60 fruits from which to choose, we limit ourselves to a half dozen, with bananas, apple juice, and grapes some of our favorite choices. Potatoes and iceberg lettuce top the vegetable list. You must drink 57 cups of apple juice to get the vitamin C in 1 cup of orange juice and eat 6 cups of iceberg lettuce to get the same amount of vitamins and minerals you could get in 1 cup of a spinach salad. In other words, we get a bigger nutritional bang for our bite by switching from apple juice to mangoes, berries, papayas, prunes, and kiwifruits, or from french fries to sweet potatoes, red peppers, broccoli, and romaine—the colorful stuff chock-full of antioxidants, vitamins, minerals, phytochemicals, and fiber.

Are You Getting Enough?
Fruits and Vegetables, That Is

Be honest. Are you religiously gobbling your daily 8 to 10 servings of fruits and vegetables? Or, are you cutting corners, fooling yourself, or even downright avoiding the produce section? Take this test and see.

1. My usual breakfast most resembles:
   a. a cup of coffee and a quick glance at the paper
   b. bacon and eggs or a Starbucks muffin
   c. a bowl of whole-grain cereal, a sliced banana, non-fat milk, and a glass of orange juice
2. My lunch typically includes:
   a. a trip through the drive-through for a hamburger, fries, and cola
   b. a sandwich, chips, and milk
   c. a low-fat entree, a tossed salad, a piece of fruit, and milk
3. My dinner vegetable is most likely to be:
   a. the thin slice of onion on my pizza
   b. potatoes, french fries, corn, and/or iceberg lettuce
   c. a dark green or yellow vegetable, a cruciferous vegetable (cabbage, broccoli, asparagus, brussels sprouts, etc.), or another deeply colored selection
4. Other than nonfat milk or soy milk, I typically drink:
   a. soda pop or coffee
   b. water, apple juice, or other fruit drinks or "ades"
   c. 100 percent fruit juice, such as orange juice, grapefruit juice, pineapple juice, carrot juice, tomato or V8 juice, or prune juice
5. At restaurants, I tend to order:
   a. steak or hamburger and fries
   b. pasta with meat or fish sauce
   c. grilled chicken or fish, a salad, steamed vegetables, and a side order of fruit

6. I order my pizza topped with:
   a. extra cheese and sausage, bacon, or pepperoni
   b. chicken or beef
   c. extra peppers, mushrooms, and other vegetables, along with a side salad
7. My normal snack during the day is:
   a. a cup of java or can of soda pop
   b. a bag of chips or a cookie
   c. baby carrots, an apple, or yogurt with berries
8. My typical after-dinner treat is:
   a. chocolate chip cookies, cake, or candy
   b. popcorn or chips
   c. berries or other fresh fruit with or without ice cream or frozen yogurt
9. On average, I include _____ vegetable(s) and/or fruit(s) at every meal:
   a. If you don't count french fries, I'm a perfect zero.
   b. one
   c. two or more

Scoring:

Answer C was your most common choice: Good work! You're probably including the recommended 8 to 10 servings of fruits and vegetables in your daily menu.

Answer B was your most common choice: You're trying to eat healthfully, but you probably are falling far short of your allotment for produce. Aim to add at least one fruit or vegetable—other than fries, iceberg lettuce, and apple juice—to each meal and snack.

Answer A was your most common choice: You've got a little work to do. You are at or below the national average of 3 servings a day. Skip the fries and include at least one citrus and one dark green leafy every day.

The latest fad diets haven't helped the fruit-and-vegetable cause. "I am afraid the current popularity of low-carb diets is encouraging people to forgo produce," Jeffrey Blumberg laments. "Who would have thought that anyone could find a way to label something that's as nutritious as fruit or carrots 'bad' for you!" Whether it's habit or the current diet trend, my son's guinea pig puts away more produce in a day than most women eat in a week.

Which Ones Are the Best?

While any unprocessed fruit or vegetable is a plus to the diet, some choices rate an A+ on the nutritional scale. Call them Mother Nature's superfoods. The following fruits and vegetables are a must in any sensible diet and help ensure health, longevity, clear thinking, and a strong resistance to colds, infection, and disease. When you accept my challenge to double your current intake of fruits and vegetables, make sure some or all of these plop onto your plate.

Dark Green Leafies

It is almost impossible to meet all your nutritional needs without including dark green leafies. A 1-cup serving of cooked Swiss chard supplies 150 mg of magnesium, or 54 percent of a woman's daily recommendation. Dark green leafies also boost your intake of fiber; vitamin C; folic acid, the B vitamin that lowers risk for heart disease, memory loss, and birth defects; vitamin K, which helps build strong bones; and the minerals calcium, iron, and potassium.

Beyond those benefits, a study from Cornell University found that of all the vegetables studied, spinach had the highest score for inhibiting cancer cells. Greens are especially good sources of the phytochemical lutein, which lowers the risk for age-related vision loss. "Generous intakes of spinach, kale, and other lutein-rich foods may reduce the risk of cataracts and macular degeneration by up to 40 percent," says Blumberg. He points out,

"People need 6 to 12 mg of lutein every day but typically consume only a fraction of that."

Green leafies are easy to include in the diet. You need at least one serving (1 cup raw or ½ cup cooked), preferably two, daily. Start by switching from iceberg lettuce to spinach in salads and sandwiches. Layer greens into lasagna; steam or chop them, and whip them into mashed potatoes; blend them with tofu for a vegetarian quiche; add them to a stir-fry; add a 12-ounce box of frozen chopped spinach to scrambled eggs, soups, or stews. Use large spinach leaves instead of tortillas to wrap around leftover meat or beans, or sauté them in a little olive oil and garlic. (Heating greens actually improves their beta-carotene and lutein content, as long as you cook them quickly in a minimal amount of liquid.)

Golden-Colored Veggies

Even a small serving of deep orange vegetables supplies five times the daily value for beta-carotene, which might lower your risk for cancer. According to Blumberg, "Diets containing 10 mg to 15 mg a day of beta-carotene (which also contain lots of other carotenoids and phytochemicals) are associated with a reduced risk of several forms of cancer." Deep orange veggies also boost defenses against colds and infections and protect the skin from sun damage. "Beta-carotene accumulates in the skin, providing partial 24-hour protection against sun damage," notes Ronald Watson, Ph.D., professor of Public Health Research at the Arizona Health Sciences Center, who adds that the more carotene-rich produce you eat, the more skin protection you get. Bright orange veggies also supply hefty amounts of vitamin C, potassium, and iron, along with more fiber than a slice of whole-wheat bread or a bowl of oatmeal.

You need at least one serving daily, preferably two, of orange-colored produce, yet Americans average the equivalent of a bite or two of a sweet potato each week. Simple ways to meet that goal abound. Microwave a halved acorn squash and top it with maple syrup and pecans. Puree cooked butternut squash and add it to soups as a thickener. Cook and mash squash to use instead of noodles or rice as a base for any dish. Use sweet potatoes instead of potatoes in salads. For golden fries, slice sweet potatoes into wedges, sprinkle on a little salt, and bake them at 425 degrees for 15 minutes. Grate carrots into spaghetti sauce, muffin batters, burritos, or tacos. Slice papayas or ruby red grapefruit to eat for snacks, add to salads, or top desserts.

Berries

Berries supply a wealth of phytochemicals, including flavonoids, caffeic acid, ellagic acid, and anthocyanins. "These compounds are potent antioxidants associated with a lower risk for heart disease and cancer, and they protect against highly reactive oxidants that damage the brain," says Gary Stoner, Ph.D., professor in the Department of Internal Medicine at Ohio State University. Berries also are high in fiber, potassium, and vitamin C and, like other fruits, help curb weight gain.

Despite their juicy sweetness, berries make it onto the menu at the rate of only about a tablespoon or two (2.1 ounces) a week. Stoner recommends including a cup of fresh or frozen berries in the diet three or four times a week. Simple ways to squeeze more berries into your diet are to toss them in salads, add them to cereal, layer them with yogurt for a parfait, heat them with Splenda and a bit of cornstarch to make a topping for waffles or desserts, and eat them frozen as an alternative to ice cream. And don't forget you can also dip strawberries in fat-free chocolate syrup, mix blueberries into salsas and blend them into smoothies, and add fresh or dried berries to muffin and pancake batters.

Kiwifruits and Mangoes

"The average woman must eat 50 percent more fruit to meet even the lower recommended limit of three servings a day," says Judith Putnam, economist at the USDA Economic Research Service, in

Washington, D.C., who tracks Americans' eating habits. One in every two women fails to get even one serving of fruit in her daily menu. Take the poor kiwifruit, for example: a typical woman eats only one chin-dribbling kiwifruit per year! We eat even fewer mangoes. The real shame is that these two fruits taste more like candy than fruit and are richer than oranges in vitamin C, packed with fiber, and a good source of vitamin A, potassium, and magnesium. Kiwifruits also are loaded with other antioxidants that help lower cancer risk and possibly stop the wheezing associated with asthma.

Eating well should be so easy! Cut a kiwifruit in half and spoon out the delicious insides, or peel it and slice it into strawberry-kiwi yogurt and serve it up with a dollop of whipped cream as a creamy dessert. Use mangoes in salsa, as a topping for fish, or in smoothies for a silky texture. Slice either fruit and drizzle lime juice on top for dessert.

Tomato Sauce

Women average less than 3 ounces of canned tomatoes daily, which is nowhere near enough. Tomatoes are an excellent source of lycopene, which is a potent antioxidant in the red pigment of plants and a possible heart saver. "Maintaining high blood levels of lycopene could lower heart-disease risk in women by up to 50 percent," says Howard D. Sesso, Sc.D., M.P.H., lead researcher on a study from Harvard that identified the heart-saving advantages of lycopene. The best place to start, he says, is to consume more lycopene-rich foods, such as tomatoes and tomato products like tomato sauce or juice. Cooked tomato products have more lycopene than fresh tomatoes. Another study suggests that lycopene also might reduce the risk for fibroid tumors, which affect up to 45 percent of women.

You'll need seven servings or more a week, each containing at least 10 mg of lycopene, which is the amount in ½ cup of tomato sauce or two fresh tomatoes. The redder the fruit, the higher the lycopene, so add vine-ripened tomatoes to salads and sandwiches, since they have more lycopene than tomatoes picked green and allowed to ripen later. Add tomato paste and sauce or canned tomatoes to soups and sauces. For a quick snack, spread tomato-based pizza sauce on a toasted English muffin, top it with low-fat cheese, and broil it until the cheese bubbles.

Produce to Avoid

While nature made all produce close to perfect, the more humans tamper with these nutritious foods, the more the health value suffers. Some foods pretend to be fruits and vegetables but really are just junk in disguise. Take a pass on the frozen waffles and pancakes with blueberries, and on the ready-to-eat cereals with apples; they typically have less than a tablespoon of fruit, and much more sugar. Likewise, fruit leathers are candy, not a serving of fruit. If you venture beyond the produce section of your grocery store, beware of the following items.

Fruit-Flavored Drinks

Anytime juice contains the wording *beverage, ade, cocktail, drink,* or *blend* in the product name, you're gulping down more sugar than nutrients. It doesn't matter if it's natural, real, or loaded with vitamins. Also, bypass any juice made from concentrated apple, pear, white grape, or a combination of these and other juices. Basically, all you're getting is highly refined sugar water, not much better than soda pop, even though the manufacturers can tout that the beverage is 100 percent juice. Dr. George Bray, of Louisiana State University, proposes that the escalating obesity rates since the 1970s coincide with increased use of high-fructose corn syrup in these beverages. Avoid the following: tangerine juice beverage, fruit juice blends, grape juice beverage, grapefruit juice cocktail, kiwi–passion fruit drink, lemonade, Hi-C, Welchade, Fruitopia, Hawaiian Punch, Sunny Delight with calcium, and, of course, Kool-Aid. Instead, quench your thirst with orange juice, grapefruit juice, prune juice, or cranberry juice. Or try flavoring water with citrus, berries, or ice cubes made from real fruit.

Fried Vegetables

The low-carb craze has diverted our attention from fat, but that doesn't mean it's safe to guzzle greasy fries, battered onion rings, or deep-fried anything. For the first time in years, our fat intake has started to climb, which has contributed to an increased calorie intake (according to the USDA, women now average 300 calories more a day than they did back in the 1980s) and weight problems, not to mention the major role fat plays in heart disease, colon cancer, and just about every degenerative disease. Instead, satisfy your cravings for crisp and crunch by choosing oven "frying," cutting up vegetables (jicamas, baby carrots, cauliflower) and dunking them in fat-free dip, and dipping apple slices in sugar-free caramel sauce.

Banana and Other Fruit Chips

Manufacturers take a perfectly healthy, fat-free banana and turn it into the nutritional equivalent of potato chips. In addition, these greasy versions of a fruit can contain trans-fatty acids, which are formed when vegetable oil is converted from a liquid to a solid during processing. These altered polyunsaturated fats act like saturated fat, raising your risk for heart disease and possibly colon cancer. Labels are now required to list the trans fat in products, so read carefully and select only foods that promise to be trans-free.

Potatoes

"One-third of our daily vegetable choices are potatoes—in particular, potato chips and french fries," says Putnam. A serving of just 10 french fries adds 158 calories and more than 8 grams of fat to the diet, much of which is artery-clogging saturated or trans fats. According to Putnam, "If you take potatoes out of the vegetable category, we are consuming very few servings of some of nature's most nutritious foods."

Switch to sweet potatoes and you'll get four times the calcium and vitamin B_2 and twice the vitamin C. While traditional potatoes have no beta-carotene, even a small sweet potato gives you three times your daily allotment of this potent antioxidant, which lowers your risk for heart disease and cancer, and reduces the redness and skin inflammation of sunburn—a sign of accelerated aging and cancer of the skin.

Salad Dressing

A plate of crispy greens is one of life's little fat-free pleasures. Not so pleasing is the fact that many fatty concoctions are guzzled under the guise of salad fixings. "Salad dressing was the number one source of fat in women's diets back in the 1990s, and with the low-carb craze, intake has probably increased since then," says Putnam. Drowning greens in dressing attests to the confusion over what is really a healthful salad and what is a fat-laden disaster. For example, a Grilled Chicken Caesar Salad at McDonald's has only 210 calories and 7 grams of fat, but add a packet of dressing and you crank the calories up to 400 and the fat to more than 24 grams (or 6 teaspoons). In a study from Pennsylvania State University, women lost weight when they started their meals with a low-calorie salad, but they ended up consuming more calories when they ate either a large or small salad packed with fatty ingredients, such as cheese and dressing.

Instead, choose fat-free dressings, or pour a small amount of dressing into a cup and lightly dip the fork into the dressing and then into the salad, leaving most of the dressing behind at the end of the meal.

Kick the Habit

How many fruits and vegetables do you need? "The Dietary Guidelines suggest each of us consume up to 13 servings of fruits and vegetables a day, with a minimum of 5 daily servings. That minimum recommendation is a very conservative recommendation," says Jeffrey Blumberg. Is five optimal? According to Winston Craig, Ph.D., R.D., chairman and professor of nutrition at Andrews University, "We don't know what an optimal dose is, but we do know that the more phytochemical-rich fruits and vegetables you eat, the more you boost your body's defenses against disease." Scratch the five-a-day minimum; aim for at least eight daily servings.

At first glance, that might seem like a lot, given that it's two to three times what most women eat. But it's really quite reasonable once you get a handle on serving sizes. A serving is:

- One small piece, such as a tangerine or plum
- A cup raw, such as strawberries
- A half cup cooked, such as applesauce
- 6 ounces of juice

If you are produce-phobic, don't give up. This is an easy habit to kick. Start small by adding just one serving daily to your regular intake, with a goal of gradually increasing fruits and vegetables until you are eating at least five, and preferably eight or more, every day. Following are other simple steps.

- **Have two at every meal.** Another simple goal in order to reach eight servings a day is to include two fruits and/or vegetables at every meal and at least one at every snack. "You must space your intake throughout the day; otherwise, you'll end up at dinner, realize you've had only an apple so far, and be faced with the daunting reality that you need seven more servings for the last meal of the day!" says Susan Moores, M.S., R.D., spokesperson for the American Dietetic Association.
- **Double up.** You don't have to eat nine different vegetables or fruits. Just double what you are already eating. For example, if you usually have a 6-ounce glass of orange juice for breakfast, increase the serving to 12 ounces and you have two servings. At lunch, a cup of spinach salad can be doubled in size, allowing you to meet the two-at-every-meal goal. At dinner, increase the ½ cup of cooked green peas to a full cup and you have two servings, for a total of six daily servings . . . and that's not even counting the apple you had for a snack and the frozen blueberries you munched after dinner.

- **Make produce superhandy.** Stock the kitchen with sturdy produce that will keep, such as sweet potatoes (which are easy to microwave), bagged lettuce (which keeps longer than loose lettuce), and bags of carrots, onions, and garlic in the crisper. Keep blueberries and orange juice concentrate in the freezer, dried cranberries or apple slices in the cupboard, and bowls of fresh fruit on the counter. Cut up fruit after dinner and place it in arm's reach, or keep a bag of baby carrots on your desk at work. "You'll be surprised how produce disappears when it is in front of you, and it's a much better choice than the chips or pretzels," says Moores.
- **Load up on veggie snacks.** Consider the produce aisle your snack aisle. Load the cart with bags of produce every time you shop.
- **Practice stealth nutrition.** Sneak fruits and vegetables into your diet:
  - Add grated carrots and zucchini to spaghetti sauce, corn to corn bread, spinach to lasagna, vegetables to canned soups, and lots of tomatoes and lettuce to sandwiches.
  - Drink your vegetables in canned tomato or V8 juice, or make your own juices either with a juicer or in the blender.
  - Please your taste buds by disguising fruit as dessert: dunk strawberries in chocolate syrup, sprinkle crystalline ginger over mandarin oranges, or mix kiwifruit into strawberry yogurt.
  - Use mashed avocado instead of mayonnaise in sandwiches. One avocado supplies a fourth of your daily need for magnesium, more than half the folic acid, a fourth of the vitamin A, and lots of B vitamins, iron, and trace minerals. While you should limit fats in general, the fats in avocados are heart-healthy while adding a rich flavor, creamy texture, and an extra dose of nutrients to meals.
- **Carry a stash.** "Always take food with you," says Debra Waterhouse, M.P.H., a registered dietitian and the author of *Outsmarting Female Fatigue*. "Stuff your purse, briefcase, backpack, gym bag, or diaper bag with apples, oranges, bananas, baby carrots, and boxes of raisins so you aren't caught

50 Ways to Love Your Fruits and Veggies

1. Mix a bag of shredded cabbage with a little light cole slaw dressing; chopped apples or canned pineapple chunks are optional.
2. Add grated carrots or zucchini to spaghetti sauce.
3. Substitute green peas for half the avocado in guacamole to reduce fat without changing the taste or texture.
4. Add chopped fresh tomatoes and cilantro to bottled salsa as a quick dip for chips, baby carrots, or pita, or pile it on as dressing for salads, tacos, and burritos.
5. Make pumpkin pie with fat-free canned milk and low-fat crust.
6. Add lots of leaf lettuce, red onion, and thick tomato slices to a turkey sandwich.
7. Pop frozen blueberries or grapes into your mouth for a sorbetlike treat.
8. Top your morning cereal with dried plums or cranberries or a handful of fresh berries.
9. Drink a travel-size box of orange juice on the way to work.
10. Stir fresh peaches or berries into frozen yogurt.
11. Add canned mandarin oranges to your spinach salad.
12. Skewer more vegetables (cherry tomatoes, carrot slices, mushrooms, eggplant, onion, squash, sweet potato, etc.) than meat on your shish kababs.
13. Add frozen green peas to canned chicken noodle soup.
14. Never, and I mean never, leave the house without a snack stash (banana, orange, apple, baby carrots, raisins, grapes, jicama).
15. Puree fresh fruit, sweeten it with concentrated apple juice, and freeze it into ice cubes or pops. Add cubes to club soda for a refreshing drink.

continued

16. Add fruit to your milkshake.
17. Make fruit or vegetable salsa and sauces with mango, papaya, peach, or pineapple and use it in place of creamed sauces on meats, fish, and chicken.
18. Sweeten nonfat, plain yogurt with fruit.
19. After dinner, place a platter of cut-up fruit on the table for snacking in the evening.
20. When eating out, order entrees that feature vegetables (grilled vegetable sandwich, salad, vegetable soup).
21. Ask your waiter to hold the potato and instead bring two side orders of vegetables (steamed) with your meal.
22. Add grapes, mandarin oranges, or cubed apples to chicken salad.
23. Skip the syrup, and top pancakes, waffles, or French toast with fresh fruit.
24. Puree vegetables such as cauliflower, carrots, or broccoli to add to soup stock and sauces.
25. Add dried fruit to stuffings and rice dishes.
26. Double your normal portion of any vegetable (except french fries or iceberg lettuce!).
27. Cut sweet potatoes into half-inch strips and roast them, for a tasty alternative to french fries.
28. Stuff an almond into each of five pitted dried plums for a sweet, chewy, crunchy snack.
29. Plan your dinner around the theme of "Meat and Three Veggies."
30. Toss a bag of frozen stew vegetables (large hunks of carrots, potato, celery, and onion) with a tablespoon of olive oil, a dash of salt and pepper, and a few sprigs of fresh rosemary. Roast at 425 degrees for 30 minutes.
31. Toss chopped tomatoes, corn, red onion, salt, and rice vinegar for a quick and filling snack or lunch salad.
32. Add cilantro, chopped tomatoes, corn, grated carrots, or other vegetables to tacos and burritos.

33. When flying, ask for tomato or orange juice for your in-flight beverage.
34. Once a week, have a meal salad for dinner, such as Cajun-salmon Caesar salad or grilled-chicken spinach salad with mandarin oranges.
35. Take advantage of precut vegetables, packaged salads, supermarket salad bars, and specialty produce.
36. Grill extra vegetables at dinner to use in a quick wrap for tomorrow's lunch.
37. Fill a halved cantaloupe with lemon-flavored yogurt.
38. Skip the fruit drinks, blends, and "ades," and go for the 100 percent orange, grapefruit, prune, pomegranate, and pineapple juices.
39. Add flowers such as dandelions, violets, daylilies, clover, and oxalis to salads.
40. Add steamed asparagus or green beans to your favorite pasta dish.
41. Top pizza with quartered artichoke hearts (canned in water), roasted red peppers, red onion, sliced zucchini, and fresh tomatoes.
42. Order deli sandwiches with extra tomatoes.
43. Whip steamed, chopped collards or chard into mashed potatoes.
44. Buy produce at various stages of ripeness to avoid spoilage.
45. Stock up on frozen plain vegetables for last-minute meals.
46. Keep dried fruit on hand for a quick snack.
47. Plant a pear or apple tree, a row of blueberry bushes, or a vegetable garden in the backyard.
48. When eating out, ask for two sides of vegetables, or split an entree and complement it with a salad.
49. At parties, sip on orange juice, tomato juice, or Bloody Mary mix.
50. Take a low-fat cooking class and share vegetable recipes with friends.

short, with the only option being a candy bar or a bag of chips from a vending machine."

What About Organic?

Choose organic foods when possible. Chemicals blanket the environment; they're on our plates and in our bodies. A study from the Centers for Disease Control and Prevention found that one in every two people tested positive for one or more of up to 116 chemicals. Other studies, however, conclude that exposure to dietary and environmental contaminants is not a serious issue, showing that unacceptable levels of pesticide residues are present in only 2 percent to 6 percent of produce samples. No one really knows how harmful pesticide exposure is for us, but to play it safe, it's wise to reduce exposure whenever possible by choosing organic foods, washing conventional produce, and eating a nutritious diet that helps strengthen the body's resistance to toxins.

Will eating organic foods lower pesticide exposure? While these foods are no more nutritious than conventional foods, studies on children who ate organically grown produce found ⅙ the concentration of pesticide by-products in the urine compared with children who ate conventionally grown produce, and a study from the University of Crete found that olive oil made from organically grown olives contained significantly lower levels of pesticides. If you can't afford organic, or if it's not available, then peel or wash produce in diluted soapy water to remove most of the pesticides.

Keep the organic issue in perspective. The thousands of studies spanning decades of research on fruits and vegetables have investigated only conventional produce, not organic, and always find health benefits. Any harm that might come from pesticides is more than overshadowed by the benefits of eating more produce.

A Dozen Ways to Eat More Fruit

1. Add chopped oranges to guacamole to make a citrusy dip for baked tortilla chips.
2. Top half a toasted bagel with cashew butter and slices of apple, banana, or mango.
3. Sprinkle pomegranate seeds over other fruits, grains, pasta salads, or tossed salads. The seeds also add zest to sauces, while the juice can be added to smoothies, ices, and salad dressings.
4. Add two kiwifruits to a 6-ounce container of strawberry yogurt. Top it with a dollop of low-fat whipped cream for a quick fruit-pudding dessert.
5. Blend any combination of fruits for a refreshing smoothie, such as chunks of pineapple, mango, and banana; vanilla soy milk, raspberries, and orange juice concentrate; or frozen mixed berries, cranberry juice, and honey.
6. Dunk apple slices in caramel sauce.
7. Add fresh cranberries to homemade apple pie.
8. Sprinkle papaya slices with a pinch of a mixture of ground cumin, cayenne, ground nutmeg, and pepper. Drizzle lime juice on top.
9. Take along a bag of fresh cherries on road trips and spit the seeds out the window.
10. Add blueberries, strawberries, or raspberries to pancake batter.
11. Mix diced peaches, apricot jam, and cinnamon to serve over French toast.
12. Snack on melon slices and low-fat cheese.

Ya Gotta Love 'em

Even die-hard produce haters learn to love fruits and vegetables. Nancy, the veggie-phobic editor who grew up hating produce, loves it now. "Today," she says, "my family eats a lot of fruit and veggies: banana or strawberry milkshakes every morning; apples, carrots, or pears at lunch; and broccoli, peas, green beans, cauliflower, spinach, or another type of green every night. And I try to have some sort of berry or melon for dessert at least three times a week—you have to serve it with a little Hershey's sauce or whipped cream, though, or it doesn't seem desserty enough!"

Setting Off Without a Plan

Lindsay, a dental assistant in Scottsdale, Arizona, is an expert on dieting. "I've tried them all," she says, "from soup-only diets to giving up anything with flour or sugar. I went totally low-fat, tried food combining, and even fasted once—I was really grumpy on that one!" She lost weight on every diet but always gained it back. Lindsay also has a family history of heart disease and wanted to avoid the mistakes her parents had made that led to health problems over the years. So, every January, she made New Year's resolutions to eat better and exercise more: "I would attack the resolution with a vengeance for the first month or so, and then by the middle of February, I was right back to my old bad habits, and the latest exercise equipment was gathering dust under the bed or in the closet."

Lindsay is hardly an exception at the dieting game. Most people swing back and forth between trying and failing to change what they eat and how much they exercise. They often blame themselves, assuming it's a lack of willpower or a fatal flaw in their characters. Blame also frequently gets placed on time, hectic work schedules, the kids, the husband, genes, the weather, the dog, you name it. None of these excuses is valid, of course. In reality, women try and fail because they are in the habit of jumping into a new diet without a realistic plan for how they will put their goals into action.

Whether we are dieting, trying to eat healthy, or determined to cut back on chips, ice cream, or doughnuts, most of us end up eating haphazardly. We start off the day with a goal to "eat less." We scrimp on breakfast and then finish off the crusts of bread on our children's plates as we clean up the kitchen, nibble off of our partner's plate when dining out, stand at the sink to polish off the chocolate cream pie before tossing the pan, or grab anything handy to quell our hunger pangs at midday. Faced with a buffet table of goodies at a party, we eat or drink more than we intended—and typically all the wrong stuff. Since memory is a poor gauge of how well we are eating, even if we review our food choices at the end of the day, most of us forget half of what we ate and minimize the faults with the rest. We don't lose weight or feel more energized, and we can't figure out why. Then we stagger into the kitchen the next morning without a plan and start the process all over again.

The habit of being planless causes big trouble. Without a plan, we just give a passing nod to our weight problems or our dreams to eat healthier. We talk the talk about wanting to drop some pounds, to exercise more, or to eat more greens. We confide to our girlfriends that we intend to cut out sugar or eat more fiber. But when it comes to walking the walk, we don't have a plan to get the job done. We might begin the latest diet or vow to eat more whole grains, but we don't sit down and formulate how we will reach that goal. The problem here is that when you don't plan what and how much you are going to eat, how you are going to eat it, and maybe even the people with whom you will eat it, you are likely to fall victim to the world around you. In this country, that means highly processed junk and a diet heavy on fat, sugar, and refined grains.

In contrast, breaking the habit by getting organized and creating a plan gives you a sense of control, self-mastery, and empowerment. A well-thought-out and simple plan can make eating right idiot-proof. A study from the University of Minnesota found that it didn't matter whether women followed low-fat or low-carb diets; what led to the greatest success was a well-thought-out, structured eating plan that included complete meals, shopping lists, and other specific tools. With that plan, even if you fall off the wagon, you know what to do. You have a structure to which to return.

That's what Lindsay found when she got off the diet roller coaster and created her own plan for eating well: "When I finally took a hard look at what I was eating and why, I realized that my problem wasn't that I needed a low-carb diet or even a low-fat diet to get my weight and health under control. I was eating too much of the wrong stuff because I wasn't leaving enough time in my schedule to prepare nutritious meals." Lindsay typically raced out the door in the morning without eating breakfast and then grabbed a drive-through breakfast burrito and coffee. She didn't pack a lunch, so she always ate with friends at restaurants. Dinner was more of the same. "I had a hundred excuses why I didn't have time," she recalls, "but the truth of the matter was I just wasn't *choosing* to make time. I was sabotaging my own efforts and didn't even realize it!"

Once Lindsay realized what was undermining her best attempts at eating right, she made a plan. "Nowadays," she states, "I put fruit, yogurt, and other goodies in a blender and refrigerate it every night. In the morning, it takes only a minute to whip up an instant breakfast that I can drink while putting on my makeup. I also get up five minutes earlier than I used to and make a quick brown-bag lunch with snacks. That's all it took to lose 10 pounds and meet my goal to eat at least five fruits and vegetables every day. Can you believe it!"

Kick the Habit

You need a specific plan to get you where you want to go. You probably wouldn't jump into the car in New York to head for California without pulling out a map to check the best route. Yet, many times, we start a diet or make a resolution without giving much thought to how we intend to reach that destination. "I vow to lose 15 pounds" or "I will cut back on sugar" are promises we make to ourselves that are so vague that there is no road map for how we will get there.

Every trip starts with the first step. "For most women, successful diet changes and long-term weight management come from modest lifestyle changes, rather than drastic measures," says Jim Hill, Ph.D., of the University of Colorado Health Sciences Center. That means simple adjustments in how you already eat and exercise. Single steps at a time, not monumental changes, are how successful plans are made.

Keep a Food Diary

Your road map to diet success begins with keeping a food journal, as discussed in Habit 1: Mindless Eating. Just logging what, how much, and when you eat, even if only for a few days, provides priceless feedback on what is getting in your way of reaching your nutrition or weight goals. "Tracking exercise and eating patterns is the most important secret to successfully creating a healthier lifestyle," says Hill. People who reach their goals and, more important, maintain the change say that keeping a food journal was their single most important strategy. Reread the "Keep a Food Diary" section in Habit 1 to refresh your memory of how to proceed.

I can guarantee that your food records will provide a few eye-openers. Maybe you'll notice that when you skip breakfast, you are likely to overeat at night, or that just keeping cookies in the cookie jar means that you grab one every time you walk into the kitchen. Perhaps your records will reveal that you eat more at dinner if you serve food family style, or that you nibble when watching television. These eye-openers are the beginning of your road map.

The next step is to create a plan to solve the problem. Maybe you decide to eat a simple, nutritious breakfast at least five days a week, or to remove the cookie jar from the kitchen counter and replace it with a bowl of fruit. Your plan might be to serve food at dinnertime only from the stove, to weigh and measure your portions before sitting down, to not go back for seconds, or to serve food on salad plates rather than larger dinner plates. Instead of eating while watching TV, you might plan to watch TV only when you're on the treadmill, or to do your nails or write letters in front of the tube so your hands are too busy to nosh.

Make the Plan Realistic

Your ultimate goal is to be the healthiest you can be. Dietwise, that means aiming for the daily guidelines set out in the Introduction, which in a nutshell are:

> 8+ fruits and vegetables
> 6 grains (3 whole grain)
> 3 calcium-rich foods
> 2 legumes, meat, chicken, fish

From there, your plan must be tailored to you, your lifestyle, and those eye-openers identified from your journal. After keeping a food diary for a few days and identifying one or two habits that block you from reaching your weight or nutrition goals, sit down and brainstorm solutions. Write down every solution that comes to mind, no matter how silly or far-fetched. If you realize that you overeat junk food at the movies, your brainstorming list could include:

- Take just enough money to get into the theater, with nothing left over to buy treats.
- Pack my own healthy snacks.
- Chew gum during the movie.
- Tie my hands together so I can't snack.
- Sit on my hands during the movie.
- Only drink water.
- Stop going to movies.

Arrange the list according to priorities, starting with the ones that contribute the most to fixing the problem, that will have the greatest impact, and that are realistic for you. Maybe you know yourself well enough to realize that you won't stop going to movies, you would be too embarrassed to tie your hands in public, and even if you have only enough money for the show, you're likely to borrow a few bucks just to have something to eat. That whittles the list down to taking along your own healthy snacks or water, sitting on your hands, and chewing gum. From there, you make a plan. A few suggestions are provided in the "Strategies, Tactics, and Tricks" section later in this chapter. Don't stop there, though. Come up with your own!

Your plan must be realistic. One of the reasons why fad diets don't work long term is that it's not realistic to expect yourself to live on cabbage soup, meals in a can, or weird food combinations for the rest of your life, let alone to expect your friends and family to tolerate that kind of change! When designing strategies, ask yourself, "Can I live with this forever? Is this a change that is relatively easy to include in my and my family's daily routine?" The best plan in the world is worthless if it doesn't fit into your life. Keep an open mind, and experiment with different strategies and tactics. The fact that one doesn't work doesn't mean you've lost the game. It just means you haven't yet found the strategy or plan that's best for you.

For Paisley, a real estate broker in Minneapolis, setting a specific plan for dieting did the trick. "I took time off from work in June," she explains, "and by July my clothes weren't fitting. So, I developed a strict five-day-a-week eating plan with two free days to splurge. If I battle a craving on a diet day, I remind myself that when the free day comes, I can have whatever I want. Usually by the time the free day arrives, I've lost the craving anyway. The plan worked. I've lost the weight, and I'm back into my clothes again."

Make sure your plan is detailed. No loopholes allowed! Let's say your problem is that you work out only once or twice a week for 30 minutes, and you want to increase that time. A vague goal to "exercise more" is bound to fail. A better plan might be to increase your workouts to four a week for 40 minutes each. That plan is easy to track. What is your road map for reaching this destination? Maybe you decide to call friends on Sunday evening and schedule four workout dates for the week, which you write in your calendar just as you would schedule a dental appointment.

Another alternative is to block out four exercise dates during your lunch hour at work.

Some people don't need a plan that is rigid. They just need a clear idea of what contributes to the problem. That was the case with Kim, a mother of three teenagers in Incline Village, Nevada, who says, "I've never gone on a diet, per se. I've watched a lot of women do it. My mother counted calories—yuk! My friends

Super Strategies

Some strategies speed the process of weight loss or better eating. For example:

- Drink nonfat milk or fortified soy milk. Not only does the calcium in milk build bones and lower your risk for colon cancer, but also, research shows that it aids in weight loss. Increasing calcium intake by the equivalent of two milk servings daily could reduce the risk of being overweight, perhaps by as much as 70 percent!
- Have soup or a salad for lunch. In studies from Pennsylvania State University, women who ate a bowl of soup or a tossed salad with low-fat ingredients for lunch cut back on calories for the rest of the meal and stayed full longer throughout the day, compared with women who ordered a casserole-type meal.
- Drink green tea instead of soda. Green tea contains caffeine and compounds called polyphenols that appear to speed the body's ability to burn fat and drop pounds.
- Snack on nuts. True, nuts are high in calories, but the fat is heart-healthy monounsaturated fat that helps with weight loss.

fasted and did Atkins and then gained the weight back. I did what made sense to me, which was eat a little less and think about what I was eating. I made small changes like smaller portions, cutting out dessert more often, eating lots of fruit and veggies, having a salad for dinner a few nights per week, and exercising more. I also started taking almonds, dried cranberries, and other healthy foods on road trips, so I didn't stop at McD's. Oh, and I took up snacking (small and healthy snacks) in between meals so I wouldn't get so hungry by mealtime. This seemed to really help the cravings, and I've been able to maintain my weight and my energy level. I can't even remember the last time I was sick!"

Your plan also is a work in progress. Some plans work; others don't. Experiment and look for a plan that fits snugly into your lifestyle. Take, for example, that exercise routine mentioned earlier. After a few weeks, add up the number of times you have exercised. If your first solution didn't work, try an evening exercise class, or go to a park where people walk and run. Measure your progress continually with stars on a calendar, check marks on a list, points on a scorecard, or whatever works best for you.

Keep in mind you are not just tracking your weight or the number of veggies consumed each day; you are tracking the *process* that affects your weight, eating, or exercise habits. Let's say your eye-opener from reviewing your food diary is that your husband brings home cookies that you can't resist. Your initial plan might be to ask him to not bring cookies home anymore (review the suggestions on how to encourage support from friends and family in Habit 2: Putting Others' Needs Ahead of Our Own). A few weeks go by, and you notice that cookies are back in the house. The first plan didn't work, so you go to Plan B, stashing the cookies someplace inconvenient, such as a cabinet that's hard to reach. Research from the University of Illinois has found that people eat what's put in front of them. The bigger the container, and the closer the food, the more they eat. They even eat more stale popcorn if it's put in front of them! "You must construct an environment that makes it difficult to mindlessly overeat big portions," says Brian Wansink, Ph.D., at the University of Illinois, Urbana-Champaign, lead researcher on these studies. He explains,

"That means divvy up packages into smaller portions, share anything that comes in an individual wrapper, and store foods away
from sight, like in the basement." After a few weeks, you might
notice that the "out of sight, out of mind" process has worked.
Great. Stick with it. If at a later date, you find yourself standing
on a chair, straining to reach those cookies on the top shelf, that
just means you need to come up with a new plan. In other words,
what works today may not work tomorrow, so stay vigilant and
creative.

Outside the Box

Your diet does not exist in a vacuum. It's part of your entire life.
You need to create a plan that embraces the bigger picture. Anne
Fletcher, M.S., R.D., author of *Thin for Life*, studied hundreds
of people who successfully maintained their weight loss. These
"masters," as Fletcher calls them, follow 10 basic strategies for
success. "Of those 10, only 3 have to do with food and exercise;
the other 7 are motivational and lifestyle strategies," says Fletcher.
Those strategies include changing your mind-set, learning to solve
your problems without turning to food, and taking control of
your life.

Sally, a graphic artist in Oregon, learned that dieting alone
wasn't the answer to making permanent changes. "I have definitely decided that weight loss is about your mind and commitment," she says, "not just what you eat. Every year, the New Year's
resolution is to diet. By January 3, I'm off it again. I finally lost
the weight for good, and the difference was my frame of mind to
really commit this time." The lesson here is that if you stick to
diet and exercise alone and don't change anything else, both in
your life and in your thoughts, it's very unlikely that you'll maintain the changes.

Information gathered from your food diary will help you identify the things that contribute to your problem with nutrition,
exercise, or weight. Maybe you realize that when you're tired, you
switch from snacking on frozen blueberries to eating a half gallon of ice cream. That means your bigger picture should include

ways to get more sleep or at least reduce fatigue. Hill points out, "If you are getting plenty of sleep, you're less likely to be irritable, stressed, or moody, and less likely to reach for fatty or sugary comfort foods." Create a plan that includes more rest or relaxation, and monitor how that change affects your health, quality of life, and eating habits. Keep experimenting with solutions until you find one or more that can solve the problem.

Your ultimate goal is to be the best and healthiest you can be. There are no Band-Aid, quick-fix solutions to achieving that goal. We all are in a continuous process of improving ourselves. Your eating or exercise habits are only part of a bigger system that also includes your thoughts and beliefs, your family's needs, social life, work hours, sleep schedule, and anything else that affects your diet and exercise. The more closely you scrutinize your lifestyle and identify factors from your food diary that contribute to bad habits, the closer you'll get to the root of your health, weight, or diet problem. Developing a plan to fix the problem is easy after that.

Two "Must-Have" Habits

While your plan will be unique and specific to your issues and life, there are two ingredients in any diet plan that are just plain essential for everyone:

- Never leave home without a food stash.
- Stock the kitchen with quick-fix ingredients for meals and snacks.

Take Food with You

You won't find baby carrots, string cheese, and soy milk at most fast-food restaurants, mini-marts, or doughnut shops. We live in a culture that Kelly Brownell, Ph.D., professor of psychology at Yale and author of *Food Fight: The Inside Story of the Food Industry, America's Obesity Crisis, and What We Can Do About It*, calls a "toxic environment." Our daily lives are virtually surrounded by fat, sugar, and calories, with no incentive to use those calories for vigorous activity.

Don't take that cultural reality as a license to splurge. Do take along your own stash. You probably wouldn't dream of leaving the house in the morning without first brushing your teeth, combing your hair, and putting on clean underwear. Well, add to that "must-do" list that you always pack a nutrition survival kit. Stash fruit, vegetables, whole-grain crackers, low-fat cheese, soy milk, salads, or whatever suits your fancy in your purse, briefcase, glove compartment, diaper bag, gym bag, or brown bag. Remember that, if you don't, you'll find yourself at the vending machine at midday choosing between a bag of chips and a candy bar.

Stock the Kitchen

Plan your kitchen. "Keep healthful staples on hand, such as pasta, frozen chicken breasts, frozen vegetables, bottled low-fat sauces, and fresh vegetables that will wait for you, such as green peppers, garlic, onions, and carrots. With a well-stocked kitchen, you can throw together a tasty and healthful meal with little or no planning," says Susan Moores, M.S., R.D., spokesperson for the American Dietetic Association.

Part of the process is first cleaning out the cupboards. Toss the unhealthy stuff, and restock with healthful foods. Use "The Healthy-Foods Shopping List" and "Revamp Your Kitchen" later in this chapter as guides for what you want to keep and what you want to toss. Even when shopping, you might need a plan, especially if you buckle under the pressure of children's demands for candy or yummy taste treats placed at eye level. Use the accompanying pointers under "Plan Ahead When Shopping" to help navigate the supermarket.

Keeping your house free of trigger foods—the ones that tempt you to eat too much of all the wrong stuff—is one way to stay on track. Are you worried about what the kids will say when you throw out the chips, soft drinks, and toaster pastries and refuse to buy more at the store? Kids can and will get all the junk they need when they're away from home, what with the car pool lady and their teachers giving them candy, and a friend's mom serving them fast-food cheeseburgers for dinner. There's no need to have this stuff in the house. You won't be depriving your kids; you'll be helping them learn good eating habits along with you.

Practice, Practice, Practice

You've settled on a plan, strategies and all. Now it's time to put know-how into practice. "The big question is 'How does a person stick with a new and healthier program year after year?' The answer to that question is that people who have been successful at any new diet habit work at it. They practice the new habits day after day. They also hook that new habit to something else that is important to them. Their walking time may be their time for spiritual reflection, or they exercise with a friend to get their daily dose of socializing," says Hill.

Any new way of dealing with food or exercise will seem a bit awkward or cumbersome at first. That's where practice comes in. Think of any skill you've learned: riding a bike, reading, driving a car, cooking, playing a sport. What did you do to acquire that skill? Practice. Practice. Practice. It took determination, patience, encouragement from friends and family, and lots of practice. "The goods news is that it gets easier with time. If people can stick with an eating and exercise program for at least two years, they are most likely to keep the weight off and sustain healthier eating habits. It's that old saying 'Practice makes perfect' put into action," says Suzanne Phelan, Ph.D., coinvestigator in the National Weight Control Registry and assistant professor of psychology at Brown University.

The Only Way to Get Better Is to Change

Planning is essential if you really are serious about getting healthy, losing weight, having more energy, or taking charge of your life. If, on the other hand, you want to stay where you are, then keep

Plan Ahead When Shopping

Careful planning can save you time, calories, and poor food choices. The following tactics are useful for making the most of grocery shopping.

- Check the cupboards, refrigerator, and your menus for the week for needed items.
- Keep a working list handy for jotting down needed items.
- Organize the shopping list according to the sections of the grocery store.
- Take advantage of advertised sales, coupons, and specials only if they are compatible with your nutrition goals.
- Never shop when hungry.
- Try not to shop with small children.
- Use a calculator to estimate the fat content of foods based on label information: multiply fat grams in a serving by 9 (calories), divide that number by the total number of calories in a serving, and multiply by 100 to get a percentage.
- Plan to be "fat content" conscious.
- Beware of marketing ploys used by grocery stores and food packagers that entice you to purchase unnecessary or unhealthy foods. Impulse items are often situated at the end of aisles, at eye level, out of place, or at the checkout stand.
- Shop primarily around the periphery of the store: the produce section, the dairy section, the bakery, and the meat department. Venture into the aisles only for real foods, such as canned beans, tomato sauce, herbs, and pasta.

right on doing what you're doing. If you're overweight, if you're inactive, or if you skimp on healthful meals, you set yourself up for premature aging, succumbing to numerous diseases, and missing out on looking great, thinking clearly, and feeling energized. If that's good enough for you, then keep doing exactly what you have been doing all along. However, the fact that you are reading this book suggests that you want more out of life. Yes, it takes a bit of work and vigilance, but that effort pays off a hundredfold. Get started on your journey by developing a plan you can live with for life.

Strategies, Tactics, and Tricks

Plans are built on strategies. Here are a few suggestions that successful weight managers and healthy eaters use all the time to help them steer their course to success.

Is your problem managing eating and the environment? Try the following:

- Sit down at a designated place, such as the dining room table, to eat.
- Eat without reading, watching TV, driving, or engaging in other activities. Chew slowly, and pay attention to flavors and textures.
- Leave food on your plate.
- Space meals and snacks so that you eat three to six times per day.
- Make temptation less visible, convenient, and available: store food out of sight; ask someone to clean up the leftovers; remove serving dishes from the table; don't bring tempting foods into the house.
- Plan another activity during eating-prone times of the day: ride a stationary bike, take a bath, polish your nails, write a letter, or walk with a friend.
- Avoid or eliminate cues that signal you to eat inappropriately. If a doughnut shop is too tempting, then take a different route to work.

- On returning home from work, go for a walk rather than enter the kitchen.
- Take nutritious foods with you whenever you go out, so you won't be enticed by the vending machine, fast-food restaurant, or cookie counter.
- Schedule "nonfood" breaks in the daily routine to visit with friends, exercise, take a warm bath, or garden.

Is your problem managing thoughts, emotions, attitudes, and beliefs?

- Avoid using food as a reward, a treat, or therapy.
- Listen to your body, and eat only when you are physically hungry.
- If you are eating in response to boredom, loneliness, or other emotions, find a way to nurture yourself that doesn't require food.
- List your beliefs about yourself and food. Replace negative beliefs that impede weight management (e.g., "Everyone must like me"; "I should be good at everything") with positive ones (e.g., "Everyone doesn't have to like me"; "It's all right to make mistakes").
- Listen to your thoughts about food and weight management. Replace negative thoughts, such as "I can't do this" or "I deserve a treat," with positive thoughts, such as "I am in charge of my weight and health" or "I've worked hard and made progress in my weight management; I won't stop now!"
- Most people have one or more problem foods that are hard to refuse, lead to overeating, or result in a slip. Plan when, where, and how much of a "trigger" food you will eat and how you will stop eating. Purchase problem foods in small quantities, and eat them only in public. Redefine problem foods as "foods I eat infrequently and in small amounts."
- Focus on what you can have, rather than what you can't have.
- Use thought stopping: visualize a stop sign in your mind whenever you catch yourself thinking a negative thought about your weight-management efforts.

Does your problem occur at restaurants and social gatherings?

- Take a vegetable platter with fat-free dip to parties.
- Surround yourself with people who support your new healthy lifestyle.
- Ask for a doggie bag at restaurants, and package half your dinner before eating.
- Eat a low-calorie snack before going to a restaurant or a party.
- Ask for gravies, sauces, and salad dressings on the side.
- Avoid alcohol, as it adds extra calories and stimulates appetite. Drink sparkling water instead.
- Decide beforehand what you will eat at a social gathering.
- Cover your plate with a napkin when you're done. (Out of sight, out of mind, and this prevents relatives and friends from pressuring you to eat more.)
- Propose a "healthful snack day" as an alternative to "dough-nut day" at work.
- Schedule business meetings at non-mealtimes.
- Encourage support by openly asking for it and modeling the type of support you would like to receive. Request that people not offer you food.

Is your problem food shopping and preparation?

- Shop from a list and never when hungry.
- Read labels to select low-fat, low-sugar foods.
- Bake, broil, steam, and dry-grill meat, chicken, fish, and vegetables.
- For the mainstay of your diet, rely on minimally processed foods, including whole grains, fresh fruits and vegetables, nonfat milk, and legumes.
- Do not cook when you're angry or anxious.
- Sip water when cooking to deter yourself from sampling the course.
- Include at least two fruits and/or vegetables at each meal and one at each snack.
- When preparing favorite recipes, use half the amount of oils, butter, margarine, and other fats.

The Healthy-Foods Shopping List

At a loss as to what to buy when switching to a healthful diet? Here's a sample shopping list with space to add your favorites. Make copies of this list to keep on the refrigerator so you can check the items you need for your next trip to the market. Or, arrange these foods to match the layout of the grocery store where you shop.

Around the Periphery

The Produce Section
___ Fresh fruits and vegetables
___ Bagged lettuce
___ Minced garlic or ginger
___ Tofu: firm, silken, regular

Extras:

_____

_____

The Bakery
___ 100% whole-wheat goods: bread, bagels, English muffins, pita, rolls, tortillas
___ Corn tortillas

Extras:

_____

_____

continued

The Dairy Case
___ Nonfat or 1% fat dairy: milk, plain yogurt, buttermilk, cottage cheese
___ Soy milk (fortified with calcium and vitamin D) or light soy milk
___ Low-fat cheeses
___ Low-fat or nonfat yogurt
___ Fat-free or low-fat ricotta cheese
___ Fat-free dairy: cream cheese, sour cream, half-and-half, whipped cream
___ Eggs or egg substitutes
___ Orange juice
___ Low-calorie margarine

Extras:

_____

_____

The Meat and Fish Department
___ Chicken or turkey breast, skinless
___ Extra-lean beef—7% fat or less by weight
___ Extra-lean pork
___ Fresh and frozen fish and shellfish

Extras:

_____

_____

The Freezer Case
___ Plain vegetables and vegetable mixes
___ Plain fruit: berries, peaches, etc.
___ Sherbet
___ Frozen fruit bars and fruit ices

___ Low-fat ice cream and sorbet
___ Orange juice concentrate

Extras:

_____

_____

Down the Aisles

Canned Goods
___ Cooked dried beans and peas ("dishes" such as chili
     or baked beans should be chosen by their fat content)
___ Tomato sauce, tomato paste, canned tomatoes
___ Low-fat marinara sauce (less than 3 grams of fat for
     every 100 calories)
___ Salsa
___ Tuna packed in water

Extras:

_____

_____

Canned and Dried Fruit
___ Fruit canned in own juices
___ Juices: orange, grapefruit, prune, vegetable
___ Dried fruit

Extras:

_____

_____

continued

Nuts, Nut Butters, and Jam
___ Nut butters: peanut, almond, soy, cashew
___ Dry roasted nuts: almonds, etc.
___ Seeds: sunflower, sesame, poppy, pumpkin
___ Jam (preferably all-fruit, no added sugar)
___ Honey

Extras:

_____

Dried Pasta and Beans Aisle
___ Dried beans and peas: kidney, black, garbanzo, navy, lima, soybeans, lentils, split peas
___ Packaged bean mixes: hummus, lentil pilaf, etc.
___ Brown rice (instant or regular), brown basmati or tex-mati rice, Wehani rice, wild rice
___ Pasta: whole-wheat, spinach, enriched

Extras:

_____

_____

Cereals
___ Hot cereals/grains: rolled oats, kasha, bulgur, quinoa, barley, other whole-grain cereals
___ Whole-grain ready-to-eat cereals: shredded wheat, Nutri-Grain, GrapeNuts, Post Whole Wheat Raisin Bran, low-fat granola, Puffed Kashi
___ Wheat germ

Extras:

_____

_____

Crackers and Cookies
___ Whole-wheat crackers: Akmak, Ry Krisp, other low-fat
___ Popcorn (air-popped)
___ Vanilla wafers

Extras:

_____

_____

Oils, Mayonnaise, and Salad Dressing
___ Fat-free or low-calorie salad dressing
___ Fat-free or low-calorie mayonnaise
___ Safflower oil, olive oil, canola oil

Extras:

_____

_____

Herbs, Spices, Nuts, and Desserts
___ Flour: whole-wheat, rye, oat
___ Herbs, extracts (vanilla, peppermint, rum, coconut, etc.), and spices
___ Sugar-free pudding mixes
___ Sugar substitutes: aspartame, Splenda
___ Baby-food prunes
___ Angel food cake mix
___ Green tea

Extras:

_____

_____

Revamp Your Kitchen

The most important of all the rules for eating well is to *always* keep your nutritional armory well stocked. Stock your kitchen, purse, briefcase, glove compartment, and/or desk drawer at work with nature's best. If you don't, you will inevitably end up at the drive-through window or the vending machine. Trust me—I've been there!

Throw out the . . .	Bring in the . . .
Whole milk	Nonfat milk or 1 percent low-fat milk
Sour cream and cream cheese	Fat-free sour cream and cream cheese
Fruited yogurt	Plain, nonfat yogurt
Cheese	Low-fat or soy cheese
Fruit drinks	100 percent fruit juice; calcium-fortified orange juice
Toaster pastries	Frozen whole-wheat waffles
Refried beans	Fat-free refried beans
Fatty cuts of red meat	Turkey and chicken breast, fish, shellfish, and legumes
Sandwich meats	Fat-free sandwich meats
Bacon	Canadian bacon
White bread and rice	Whole grains
White flour	Whole-wheat flour
Flour tortillas	Fat-free, whole-wheat, or corn tortillas
High-sugar cereals	Oatmeal, wheat germ, and whole-grain cereals

Granola	Whole-grain nugget cereals
Butter	Olive oil
Hard margarine	Soft tub margarine
Shortening	Pureed fruit, such as apple butter or baby-food prunes, for baking
Mayonnaise	Low-calorie or fat-free mayonnaise; gourmet mustards
Salad dressing	Fat-free vinaigrette
Fatty dip	Boxed or premade hummus; black bean dip
Heavy-handed saltshaker	Fresh herbs; lemon juice; red pepper flakes; garlic
Hoisin sauce	Ginger
Iceberg lettuce	Leaf lettuce, spinach, and romaine
Convenience snack items	Fresh fruits and vegetables
Fruits canned in heavy syrup	Fresh fruit and fruits canned in their own juice
Frozen vegetables in sauce	Plain frozen vegetables
Soda pop	Water, soy milk, and fruit juice
Potato chips and corn chips	Nuts, seeds, and dried fruit
Doughnuts and pastries	Whole-wheat bagels
Ice cream	Sorbet; fat-free frozen yogurt; frozen blueberries or grapes; all-fruit Popsicles
Chocolate fudge	Cocoa; fat-free fudge sauce; fat-free chocolate syrup

Excuses, Excuses, Excuses

"I've tried every diet, and I just can't lose weight. It must be my metabolism."

"I want to exercise; I really do. I just don't have time."

"Both my mother and sister are heavy. There's no diet that will work for me. I inherited this 'pudge'!"

"I can't afford to eat healthy. Do you know how much a mango costs!"

"I gained weight with each baby, and that type of weight never comes off."

"I would eat healthy, but my family would never go for it."

"I have no willpower, so I am destined to be fat."

"Exercise makes me hungry, so I eat more and gain weight. I can't win."

"I don't like vegetables, so eating better is pretty much out of my league."

"Diets don't work. Everyone just gains back the weight. Why bother?"

"I don't eat dairy products because I'm allergic to milk."

"I'd eat better, but health food tastes like cardboard."

"I gain weight just looking at a cheeseburger. Guess I was just born to be heavy."

We are masters at the habit of making excuses and shifting blame. We assert that we want to eat well, but in the same breath we lament how hard it is to find the time, money, and know-how to make it happen. Our reasons, rationales, claims, arguments, and justifications run the gamut. Eating well is inconvenient, or it gives us gas. Our friends will make fun of us, or we're ruled by a sweet tooth. We're sure that what's undermining our best intentions is our glands, our hormones, our lack of time, our uncontrollable cravings, or, when all else fails, our husbands, partners, kids, parents, friends, work, school, or dog—unless it's the weather. We blame our sugar cravings on PMS, our need for chocolate on biology, our love handles on that leftover pregnancy weight, and an inability to keep our spoons out of the ice cream on stress. If it weren't for our lives, eating well would be a snap!

"For years, I used school as an excuse for why I couldn't drop weight," says Paisley, a real estate broker in Minneapolis. "I was so preoccupied with studying and meeting deadlines that I grabbed food when I could, drank too much coffee, and ate too-large dinners every night. Once I graduated, I couldn't use that excuse anymore and was forced to face the reality that it was I, not school, that had packed on the excess weight."

You Can Change

Many women develop the mind-set that it's simply impossible to eat well. But people do change every day despite overwhelming odds. Of the 71 million of us dieting and the many more who just want to eat better, about one in every five will actually make the necessary changes to maintain weight loss for good; even more make simple dietary changes that yield profound benefits to their health.

How do those success stories do it? They get real. That's what both the National Weight Control Registry (NWCR), an ongoing research study based at Brown University, and Anne Fletcher, M.S., R.D., author of *Thin for Life*, independently found as they studied people who had lost an average of 60 pounds and maintained the loss for more than a year. For these "masters" to achieve what they did, it didn't matter whether they were heavy as kids, how many times they'd dieted in the past, or how they finally lost the weight, according to Suzanne Phelan, Ph.D., coinvestigator in the NWCR and assistant professor of psychology at Brown. "This time, something clicked for these people," Phelan says. "For the first time, they gave up the excuses and were thoroughly committed to change their behaviors, lose weight, and be physically active."

The deciding moment for many success stories was when they realized that the process of eating well or of losing weight and keeping it off was up to them. They had to stop blaming everything from their genes to their kids and take responsibility for their lives. "People failed at past dieting attempts because they weren't losing weight for themselves," says Fletcher, "but rather for the spouse, the parents, or someone else. Once they realized that there was no magic bullet and that the buck stopped here, they accepted that managing their weight problems and their diets was entirely up to them and was a lifelong process within their power." They decided the changes they must make for life were worth it for themselves, their health, their well-being, and their self-respect. As a result, they dropped the "why me?" mantra. They stopped making excuses for why they didn't exercise or why they just didn't have time to eat well.

As discussed in earlier chapters, many women are their own worst enemies when it comes to making diet changes or losing weight. They want to be healthier, have more energy, think faster, look younger, and be thinner, but they give up the power to make those changes by putting the blame for not reaching those goals on something or someone else. That's not news to Vince Nistico, M.S., an ACE-certified (American Council of Exercise) personal trainer in Salem, Oregon, who relates, "New clients often complain about their weight, but their response to even my most benign suggestions to increase their activity level, such as take the stairs or park farther away, is an emphatic 'I tried all that, and none of it worked.' What they're saying is that they really want to look and feel better, but at the same time they are determined to sabotage their own efforts."

Kick the Habit

What are your excuses? Everyone has them. If a few don't jump to mind immediately, try this: Say to yourself, "I will start a diet tomorrow." Now listen to the tiny voices in your head as they start churning out reasons why you can't, such as "Not now; I'm too busy," "I'll have to wait until after the party this weekend," "I can't go on a diet because my husband insists on eating out twice a week," or "I can't give up my afternoon chip fest."

There are simple ways to get by those automatic roadblocks and never look back. Kick the excuse habit forever by taking charge of your life, your diet, and your exercise. Let's bust a few excuses and bask in tried-and-true solutions.

It doesn't matter what I eat or how much I exercise; I can't lose weight because I have a slow metabolism.

The vast majority of women who are overweight have normal metabolisms, so they can't blame their waistlines on their glands. Yet, some people seem to put on the pounds by just looking at food, while others can indulge now and again with no worries. "It is unclear whether genetic or environmental differences are the reason people handle calories differently," says Robert H. Eckel, M.D., professor of medicine at the University of Colorado Health Sciences Center and chair of the American Heart Association's Council on Nutrition, Physical Activity, and Metabolism. Maybe their enzymes (such as lipoprotein lipase, or LPL) that aid in fat burning are less efficient, or maybe they burn fewer calories in maintaining body heat. Maybe their leaner friends just expend more calories fidgeting. Whatever the reason, some people naturally store a little bit more as fat when they overeat.

Even if you are genetically inclined to be chubby, you still can be leaner or healthier by eating right and exercising daily. Diet successes in the NWCR have proved that. Many subjects were overweight as children; still more had tried diet after diet in the past, to no avail. When they finally got serious about taking charge of their health, that's when they dropped the weight and kept it off. "Those people who have a slower metabolism just need to increase their exercise to make up the difference," says John Foreyt, Ph.D., director of the Behavioral Medicine Research Center at Baylor College of Medicine and an expert on weight management.

I inherited my "pudge" from my mother, and there is nothing I can do about it.

Yes, parents pass on their eating and exercise habits, as well as their genes. However, before you attribute your waistline to your ancestors, consider that up until a generation or two ago, few people were overweight. Studies show that up to 85 percent of a person's eating habits are learned, not inherited. In short, genes probably are not the reason why people are gaining too much weight today.

It takes thousands of years to tweak our DNA, so our genes are virtually the same as cave dweller Jane's forty thousand years ago. "Escalating obesity is a phenomenon of the past few decades and reflects a head-on collision between our ancient genes and our current lifestyles," says Tom Baranowski, Ph.D., professor of behavioral nutrition at Baylor College of Medicine. Genetics may increase your susceptibility to obesity, but those ticking genes explode into a weight problem only with the help of habits. Studies show that people who finally succeed at permanent weight loss often come from families in which being overweight is the rule. The mother, father, sisters, and brothers are all overweight, and so were they until they broke the mold and lost the weight for good.

What about that set point you've heard about? The set point theory states that whenever your weight falls below an internal standard, your metabolism adjusts, slowing down to use fewer calories, thereby making you resistant to weight loss. The flaw in this theory is that if your metabolism really worked this way, you'd also resist weight gain, because your metabolism would rev up to bring you back to your standard weight. "I prefer the term 'settling point' to set point," says Eckel, who explains that we all are preprogrammed to weigh a certain amount, but the environment determines where our weight settles. By far the biggest difference between your weight and the next woman's comes more from what you eat and how much you move. Some people may never be skinny, but everyone can lose weight and be healthier!

I don't have time to exercise.

My guess is you do have the time; you just need to see where you're wasting it. Take an honest look at how you spend your day, by keeping an activity log. Write down what you do hour by hour for a few days, including weekend days. You'll be surprised how much time you spend sitting around, staring out the window, or watching television. Then, ask yourself where you can fit in two or three 10-minute walks or exercise breaks each day.

Without exercise, you can't reach your health goals. That lazy little devil in your head might rant and rave about how you don't have time, but you have to ignore those excuses and find time. No diet alone will prevent premature aging, improve your mood, sharpen your thinking, or cure a host of other ills; you must also become a convert to daily physical activity.

Other Excuses That Roadblock Success

- **I'm allergic to dairy foods.** Skipping milk skews the odds in favor of not getting enough calcium and vitamin D, two nutrients essential in the prevention of osteoporosis and colon cancer. Less than 3 percent of the population is allergic to milk products; however, many more have an inability to digest milk sugar, a condition called lactose intolerance. Even then, most can tolerate a half cup of nonfat milk with meals. Other alternatives are lactose-treated milk and soy milk fortified with calcium and vitamin D.
- **Beans give me gas.** Don't miss out on one of Mother Nature's best sources of fiber, iron, zinc, protein, B vitamins, and health-enhancing phytochemicals that lower heart disease and cancer risk. Rinse canned beans under running water to remove raffinose and stachyose, the two sugars that cause gas. Add small amounts of beans to soups and salads, to allow your

body to adjust. Or, use Beano, a natural product that counteracts gas formation.

- **I hate fish.** Give fish another chance. You'll be giving yourself the best source of the omega-3 fats that lower the risk for heart disease, dementia, depression, osteoporosis, and more. Try delicate-flavored types, such as snapper, flounder, and trout. Buy very fresh fish, since the "fishy" smell is a sign that seafood has been lying there for a while. If you still can't stomach fish, consider taking fish oil supplements.

- **I'm too tired to exercise.** Exercise in the morning, before you crash or find distractions from exercise. Eat breakfast and drink water, so you'll have more energy all day long. Combine carbs and protein at lunch, such as a turkey sandwich, to keep you satisfied and energized throughout the afternoon hours. Also, watch your sugar intake, since sweets might pick you up temporarily, but they'll drag you down later in the day.

- **I can't exercise because I have a bad shoulder, knee, back, ankle, wrist, elbow. . . .** There is always some form of exercise for everyone, no matter what the handicap. Don't let this lame excuse stop you from getting on with your life!

- **I'm gaining weight because I'm getting older.** Wrong. Research shows that women gain about a pound a year after age 30, but not because metabolism slows. It's lack of exercise and loss of muscle that slows metabolism. A combination of aerobic and strength-training activity is all you need to boost metabolism.

- **I gained weight with each baby.** Exhaustion and convenience lead new mothers to rely on quick-fix packaged foods and grazing on junk. A study from the University of Texas found that women are most likely to gain weight after the baby is born if they stop exercising, eat high-fat foods, and have a poor body image.

I've tried exercise, and I didn't lose weight. In fact, I gained weight!

If you add daily semivigorous exercise to your routine and keep your food intake steady, you will lose weight. You'll lose even more when you reduce your food intake. If you don't lose weight, you are either overestimating how much you exercise, underestimating how much you eat, or defying the laws of physics. More than likely, it's a blend of the first two. Never is it the last.

Research shows repeatedly that the heavier a women is, the more she overestimates how much exercise she gets. Researchers at the University of Alabama conclude that if most women were moving as much as they thought, they'd burn almost a thousand more calories a day. In the study in question, women reported how much physical activity they got while cleaning, gardening, climbing stairs, and walking. All the women overshot their exertion levels, but the heaviest subjects overestimated by about 900 calories, while leaner women overestimated by an average of 600 calories. The problem is that if women already think they are physically active, there is no reason to do more. "People consistently underestimate their food intake and overestimate their activity, so I recommend that they keep journals and then add at least a third more calories from food and cut about the same in their estimated activity," says Foreyt. (For details on accurately measuring your food and exercise, refer to Habit 3: Not Being Honest.)

Another miniexcuse might be at the root of this excuse. Women often rationalize a pig-out session by saying, "I exercised; therefore I can eat." Shelve that excuse immediately! You can easily gain weight with exercise if you more than make up the difference in cupcakes! "If I can't overeat after a six-hour training ride, no one can," says Omer Kem, professional cyclist for Team Subway.

Of course, this excuse also might really be a cover-up for a less-than-excited attitude about exercise. Not everyone falls in love overnight with sweating. Expect ups and downs, stops and starts, with any exercise program. With time and persistence, working out should become easier and more enjoyable. If not, do it anyway. People are most likely to stick with an exercise routine if they do it in the morning before a host of other activities and obligations compete for their time. Don't give yourself the opportunity to ask, "Should I go to the gym today?" Chances are you won't. Quit agonizing and just go.

I don't have time to eat well.

Time is your archenemy. Do you say that you would willingly eat better if only you had the time? What if I told you I'd pay you $200 for every healthy meal you eat? Would you find the time then? If so, then time isn't the issue; prioritizing is.

The first place to check is the television. If the only thing most women were to do is cut back on a few hours of television viewing, they probably would have more than enough time to fix three square gourmet meals a day. The average woman spends 5 hours a day, 34 hours a week, watching television. That's almost the equivalent of a full-time job! Research shows that for every two hours of TV viewing, the risk for being overweight increases by 23 percent and the risk for diabetes increases by 14 percent. TV watching slows our metabolism more than any other activity except sleeping. It encourages binge eating, exposes us to an onslaught of junk-food commercials, and even puts a damper on our moods.

Besides, it doesn't take much time to eat well, especially with the wealth of new, healthful convenience foods. You don't need to eat a hot meal or even cook in order to be healthy. With a well-stocked kitchen, it takes less time to prepare a low-fat, nutritious meal than it does for that take-out order to arrive. It does take a change in mind-set and a little planning up front. For example:

- **Keep nutritious foods readily available.** Clean and store enough raw vegetables to supply meals and snacks for up to three days. (Or purchase vegetables, salad greens, or fresh fruit already washed and cut.) Freeze an extra loaf of whole-wheat bread; stock extra cans of kidney beans; fill the cookie jar with homemade trail mix made with nuts, dried fruits, roasted soybeans, and a few chocolate chips.

Get Moving!

No more excuses. Your health and your waistline depend on both a good eating plan and exercise. Here are the steps to take to get moving.

1. Ask yourself why you want to exercise. Don't be vague, with answers like, "Because it's good for me." Spell out your reason. For example, "Exercise will help me shave two inches off my waist, think more clearly, have more energy, meet new people, lower my blood cholesterol, lower my blood pressure, help me sleep, lift my PMS blues, make me sexier, and lower my diabetes risk."
2. List all your excuses for not exercising. Then counter each excuse with either a plan to overcome that obstacle or a reason why it's not valid.
3. List activities that suit you, your time constraints, and your lifestyle.
4. Set goals, and establish ways you will reward yourself for each accomplishment. Again, be specific. A goal might be, "I will walk briskly (play tennis, snowshoe, take an aerobic dance class, etc.) three days a week for 45 minutes each time and will lift weights at the gym (in the living room, in the hotel fitness club, etc.) for 30 minutes two days a week."
5. Keep an exercise log to monitor your progress.
6. Reward yourself with stars on a calendar for days when you exercised, a favorite TV show, a movie, or new clothes.

• **Make more than you need.** When preparing a meal, cook extra chicken or brown rice, chop extra celery or green onions, grate extra carrots, or squeeze extra lemon juice, and store it in the refrigerator to use later in the week.

- **Prepare meals in quantity.** Make a big pot of soup or stew, spaghetti, lasagna, casseroles, chicken or bean wraps, or sauces that are great for lunches or dinners throughout the week, or to freeze in individual containers for later consumption.
- **Keep it simple.** Unless you are a gourmet cook who loves to spend hours in the kitchen, avoid complicated recipes that require considerable time, a lengthy list of ingredients, and fancy equipment.
- **Take advantage of nutritious quick-fix foods.** Purchase pre-cut vegetables and fruits, bottled minced garlic or ginger, bottled lemon juice, frozen whole-wheat waffles, shredded cabbage, bagged lettuce or spinach, bulk bags of frozen skinned and boned chicken breasts, canned kidney beans, and ready-to-eat hummus.
- **Maximize your options.** Don't waste time and calories on nutritional duds. Choose mostly colorful fruits and vegetables, water, whole grains, nonfat and plain-milk products, legumes, fish, poultry breasts, olive oil, and nuts.

As for that TV watching, count on gaining weight if you watch two hours or more a day. It's to your advantage to eat dinner at the table and finish before turning on the TV. Knit, do needlepoint, or, better yet, ride the exercise bicycle instead of eating when the TV is on. Better still, unplug the TV twice a week and devote the time to family, exercise, and other healthy habits.

I've tried everything, and nothing works.

Everyone's plan for eating healthy and managing weight is different. What works for one woman might not work for another. That doesn't give you license to give up. So, you tried and failed when you gave up butter on your toast, walked a half hour a day, took a supplement, hired a personal trainer, or any of thousands of other dieting tricks. First, ask yourself if you truly did try the last time or if you gave it a halfhearted effort and then quit. Second, ask yourself what the reasons were for your not succeeding the last time. Perhaps your diet attempts coincided with a job change, which upset a plan that might work just fine now that

No Time? Here Are Nine 10-Minute Dinners

- Grilled chicken breast topped with bottled salsa and steamed frozen carrots. Dessert: Fresh pineapple cubes sprinkled with sugar, chopped mint, and chopped pine nuts.
- Canned lentil soup with a slice of bread, low-fat cheese, and apple slices. Dessert: Mango slices sprinkled with chili powder and drizzled with lime juice.
- Bagged lettuce topped with precooked chicken, canned black beans, and sliced red onion. Dessert: Store-bought angel food cake topped with berries.
- Take-out pizza topped with extra tomato slices and served with bagged baby spinach. Dessert: Peach slices and blueberries drizzled with a mixture of honey, lemon juice, and lemon peel.
- Spread mustard on a slice of whole-wheat bread. Top it with a thick slice of tomato and a thin slice of low-fat cheese. Broil it until the cheese bubbles. Serve your open-faced sandwich with orange slices and baby carrots. Dessert: A cup of fat-free cocoa.
- Make mac and cheese from a box (skip the butter/margarine). Mix in cooked chopped frozen broccoli or spinach (fresh or microwaved from frozen). Or, top it with tomato slices and brown it in the broiler. Dessert: Frozen blueberries.
- Fill a heated tortilla with drained canned black beans, grated low-fat cheese, leftover vegetables, and salsa. Roll it up and top it with a teaspoon of fat-free sour cream. Dessert: Peach sorbet sprinkled with cinnamon sugar.
- Cook pasta. Toss it with commercial pesto sauce and precooked shrimp. Serve with a bagged-lettuce salad. Dessert: Drained canned mandarin orange segments topped with crystallized ginger.

- Frozen entrees: Weight Watchers Smart Ones Swedish Meatballs, Lean Cuisine Chicken Parmesan, or Healthy Choice Grilled Turkey Breast. Serve it with steamed frozen vegetables and a glass of soy milk. Dessert: Fresh strawberries dunked in fat-free chocolate syrup.

life has settled down. If you feel that you really did try, all that means is either you haven't yet found the right solution for you or something caused you to slip from your program, and that slip quickly progressed to a relapse.

When it comes to changing habits, especially diet and exercise habits, everyone gets tripped up, makes mistakes, and falls off the wagon. It's jumping back on that separates the successes from the failures. "People who have lost weight and, more important, kept the weight off attack slips quickly. At the first sign of even small increases in weight, they immediately return to the plans and strategies they used to lose the weight in the first place," says Suzanne Phelan. Anne Fletcher found the same pattern with her masters. One of their 10 keys to success was nipping a setback in the bud. (More on how to handle slips is provided in Chapter 10: The All-or-Nothing Approach to Dieting.)

Don't roll over and play victim. Stop blocking your road by stubbornly insisting that you've tried everything and nothing works. Keep trying until you find the right mix of habits that will bring health and vitality to your life. Give it your all-out commitment. I promise it's worth the effort!

I can't afford to eat healthy foods.

Nice try, but no go. With a little planning, eating well can actually cost less than typical fast-food fare. A study from the Research Institute at Bassett Health Care, in Cooperstown, New York, found that following a heart-healthy diet reduced a person's shopping bill by up to $8 a week. For a family of four, that could mean about $1,664 in annual savings. Dietitians at the "5-a-Day" program also made a few healthful changes in a typical menu and saved almost $1 a day.

I'm not denying that wild salmon and imported olive oil cost more than a fast-food supersaver meal, but don't discount the hidden costs of a bad diet. "Supersized portions of cheap food appear to be a great deal until you factor in the added costs of wardrobes, weight-management programs, health care, and lost days of work due to complications of being overweight; then it's not such a bargain," says Barbara Rolls, Ph.D., of Pennsylvania State University. More than one in every two of us is eating too much, with the extra pounds costing a person more than $5,000 in added health-care bills, plus the more than $33 billion spent annually in this country on weight-loss products and services. All of a sudden, that supersaver meal isn't so cheap.

You don't need to go broke to eat well. After all, pound for pound, health-boosting oatmeal, beans, and apples are a lot cheaper than eggs and bacon, steak, or even chips. To pare down the food bill, try these approaches:

- Buy the less expensive produce such as apples, oranges, carrots, and cabbage.
- Look for specials and use coupons.
- Buy in bulk items such as oatmeal, rice, nuts, and staples; shop at warehouse clubs for better bargains on larger quantities.
- Switch from meat to beans, which are much less expensive.
- Take food with you so you're not tempted to make impulse purchases of expensive items.
- Buy generic or store brands of frozen vegetables, canned fruit, milk, and other items that typically cost less than brand names.

I have no willpower.

Let's burst this bubble right away. Willpower is not something you either were born with or were not. In fact, there really is no such thing as willpower. Resisting temptation isn't a matter of inner strength; it's about learning and practicing new habits, which also is what this book is all about. Try visualizing yourself resisting temptation, as a form of practice with no risk of giving in to the food. Find a quiet place, close your eyes, and imagine yourself faced with an enticing food, such as chocolate, and successfully avoiding the temptation.

Another solution to breaking this habit is to control your environment. Take the example of a half gallon of ice cream: You don't need willpower to keep from eating the whole thing—you need practical steps for controlling your surroundings. That means creating an environment conducive to success. For example, keep ice cream out of the house, fill up on healthier food so you are not hungry, or find nonfood ways to curb the stress that underlies your temptation in the first place. (The following chapter delves further into food and mood.)

I don't need to change my diet, because I'm already healthy (or, I don't need to exercise—chasing the kids around is all the activity I need).

Only one in every 100 people meets even the minimum standards of a balanced diet. Not even 20 percent of us exercise enough. You might be one of those rarities, but even then there is always room for improvement. "One big mistake people make is confusing eating a few healthy foods with eating an overall healthy diet," says Susan Moores, M.S., R.D., spokesperson for the American Dietetic Association. Add an apple to a meal of a cheeseburger, fries, and a cola, and you haven't made up for the glut of saturated fat, calories, and salt in that meal. When it comes to being active, the fatigue you feel after a day of chasing kids is mostly mental exhaustion, not a real workout.

Being overweight or having obvious signs of disease are not the only criteria for making healthful changes in your diet. Besides, most of us are at risk for disease and don't even know it. Most women after age 35 have blood pressure or cholesterol levels above normal and are at future risk for disease. Optimal levels are lower than normal, so a blood pressure reading should be

I Just Can't Motivate Myself!

Do you have a problem staying motivated? Take a run at these stick-with-it tricks.

- Reward yourself frequently—with something other than food. Place tally marks on a calendar, tokens in a jar, or money in a piggy bank each time you accomplish a ministep. Use the "If . . . then" rule: for example, "If I eat five servings of vegetables and fruits today, then (and only then) I will go to a movie tonight."
- Remember this motto: If you don't like the way you are feeling, change the way you are thinking.
- Team up with a friend. You'll be much more likely to adhere to your diet or exercise plan if someone is counting on you.
- Join a gym, hire a trainer, participate in a support group, or enroll in a healthy-cooking class.
- Surround yourself with reminders to eat well and exercise. Place your gym bag next to your desk at work, post a "When will you exercise today?" sign on the fridge, keep a bowl of baby carrots on your desk.
- Identify your slip-prone situations, from negative thoughts to a change in routine, and plan how you will handle them.
- Give yourself credit for daily successes.
- Visualize yourself ahead of time successfully handling risky food issues and social situations.
- Recognize that changing habits will require an initial investment of time.
- Focus on gradual lifestyle changes and not on dieting or weight loss.

less than 120/80, and a blood cholesterol level should be less than 200 mg per deciliter. Even if you have optimal levels, you can't close the book on making changes: most women in the optimal category move on to "normal" and then to "high normal" and then to "high" as they get older.

Prevention is much more effective than treatment. For example, a woman who has high blood pressure or cholesterol, even with medication, is twice as likely to have a heart attack or stroke as a woman who never had elevated levels. Don't wait until you enter the high-risk group to get a diet move on. "The sooner women make healthful changes in their diet, the greater the benefits to their health today and in the future," Moores asserts.

My family will never agree to healthy eating.

Do you find yourself pointing the finger at your kids or your partner to account for your failure to eat more healthfully? That's what Sally, a graphic artist in Bend, Oregon, did. She admits, "Cooking for my husband and kids was one excuse I used for years to explain why it was OK for me to eat 'normally,' which meant too much. I explained to myself that my family just wouldn't want to eat the way I knew I should, so I put things off." She continued to bring hot dogs and doughnuts into the house, she says, using the excuse that the kids liked those goodies: "But I was the one who ate most of them! I'd plan to shed the pounds after my birthday; then after Easter; then after the kids got out of school. When all else failed, my excuse was that I didn't have the money to join Weight Watchers. There was never the perfect time to start eating right."

Women are the primary gatekeepers for food coming into the house. What we buy and prepare is pretty much what our families eat. Yeah, they might gripe a bit when we switch from corn dogs and fries to grilled chicken and broccoli, but never do children die of starvation in a house full of food. They not only adapt but also learn healthy eating habits that will last a lifetime. A study from the University of Minnesota found that children who sat down to healthy family dinners were less likely to smoke, use alcohol or drugs, battle depression, or attempt suicide, and were more likely to maintain high GPAs. A study from Fred Hutchinson's Cancer Research Center, in Seattle, found that a woman's diet was the biggest predictor of what her husband ate. When women adopted low-fat, healthful diets, the men's diets improved, too. Their calories, cholesterol, and fat intake decreased, and both spouses lost weight. You'll be doing your family a huge favor by eating better.

Take Responsibility

There is no excuse too imposing for not eating well and exercising more. Every excuse can be overcome. That is, except for your own belief that you can't do it. Change your attitude and you change your life. Experts, such as your physician, a personal trainer at the gym, or a therapist, can offer advice. Friends and family can provide support. But no one but you can take responsibility for yourself. No magic pills, no diet gurus, and no gizmos or gadgets can do it for you. The women who succeed at making healthful changes in their lives are the ones who put aside the habit of making excuses and take it upon themselves to change their behaviors, for good.

I'm Moody—Let's Eat!

"It was a harmless plate of chocolates. Why did they beckon to me? I tried to ignore them, even left the room, but it was no use. I felt like some kind of addict, needing my chocolate fix. I waved good-bye to my willpower, and there I was, eating one and then another and another. I couldn't stop. No matter how many pieces I ate, I didn't get full. I wasn't even hungry: why did I keep eating?"

Sharon, a fitness instructor in San Diego, sat in my office angry and frustrated with herself. She'd not lost the 2 pounds that had been her goal that week, and she was sure it was because her husband had brought home that box of candy. She couldn't understand why she'd eaten so many. She hadn't planned to do it. In fact, she'd planned to not eat chocolate all week. Why did she throw all caution to the wind and eat half the box?

That's not an easy question to answer. There are almost as many theories about what governs appetite and triggers out-of-control eating as there are enticing foods on grocery shelves. "We have a lot to learn about appetite and satiety, and it's likely we'll find in the long run that the underlying reasons why people overeat are a combination of factors," says Barbara Rolls, Ph.D., professor of nutrition at Pennsylvania State University.

Even the definition is tricky. Hunger, or the inborn instinct to eat, is a facet of appetite. But if hunger were all that mattered, then eating would be a simple matter of feeling physiological hunger, seeking food, eating in response to that need, and pushing back from the table at the first sign of fullness.

That doesn't explain Sharon's uncontrolled reaction to the box of chocolates. Obviously, many of us sometimes eat more than we need, whether we're hungry or not, and often all the wrong stuff. Sometimes what leads us astray is our brain chemistry—a symphony of appetite-control chemicals, including serotonin and the endorphins. Other times, we eat for emotional, not physical, reasons, such as when we are angry, stressed, anxious, lonely, scared, happy, excited, or bored. Janet, a freelance writer in Carlsbad, California, is a perfect example. "I admit it," she proclaims, "I'm an emotional eater. I eat when I'm down in the dumps, lonely, feeling sorry for myself, you name it. I turn to food for solace, and my food of choice is ice cream; make that chocolate ice cream!" Janet's wake-up call came, she says, when her cholesterol levels started to climb: "I'd been so healthy up until that point. It was a real shock, one that got me motivated to take better care of myself."

Still other times, we eat because the food is there, because others are eating, because that's what you are supposed to do at lunchtime, because it smells or looks good, or because we don't want the food to go to waste. Jenny, an occupational therapist in Corvallis, Oregon, says, "I hardly ever eat because I'm really hungry. More often than not, I eat because the food is there—because it looks good or smells good." As cited earlier in this book, in his research on what leads people to eat too much, Brian Wansink, Ph.D., at the University of Illinois, Urbana-Champaign, found that merely placing food in front of people or giving them big servings is enough to cause overeating. Put women in front of a movie screen and give them popcorn, and you have the perfect setup for overeating. Mood just adds insult to injury—women eat even more if the movie is a tearjerker. In short, giving an upset woman something tasty primes her for an all-out splurge. There is a physiological reason why we eat when upset: the food calms us down.

That's what turned out to be the case with Sharon. As I continued to question her about the events directly preceding her chocolate binge, she commented that the day had been unusually stressful. She'd had a fight with a coworker, a participant in one of her classes had tripped and twisted an ankle, and the drive home had been a nightmare. "I walked in the door with my head pounding and my shoulders up around my ears," she moaned. That could explain why she took one look at the chocolates on the kitchen counter and dived in with a vengeance.

"The number one predictor of diet relapse is emotional issues, especially stress," says John Foreyt, Ph.D., director of the Behavioral Medicine Research Center at Baylor College of Medicine. According to Foreyt, "Anytime your feelings get in the way, you're likely to lose control of your eating." Women are quick to adopt the habit of soothing mood with food. When the going gets rough, we are much more prone than men to crave foods, to use food to help ourselves feel better, and to overindulge in sweet-and-creamy comfort foods, such as ice cream and chocolate. We eat to celebrate, to commiserate, to wake up, and to wind down. Turning to chocolate to mend a broken heart or calm rattled nerves only adds stress to your life by packing on the pounds and pulling the rug out from under you in your pursuit of eating well. This is not a habit you want to encourage!

Food for Solace or Sustenance?

Our minds and moods thrive on a certain mix of fuels. What and when we eat, even at a single meal, can affect whether we feel happy, sad, irritable, alert, or sleepy. Certainly, abrupt mood swings sometimes can be symptoms of serious medical conditions, but more often than not, the foods we eat are the culprit. For example, Sharon might feel energized after eating chocolate, mainly because the sweet rush temporarily increases blood sugar, but the crash that follows the high is usually worse than the feeling that prompted her to reach for those treats. Other times, skipping breakfast may leave you feeling fine for an hour or two, but your appetite-regulating chemicals soon spiral out of control, leading to dwindling energy, poor concentration, and food cravings by midmorning. "On the other hand, eat the right foods at the right time, and you'll be amazed at how good you feel, how clearly you think, and how much easier it is to manage your weight," says Debra Waterhouse, M.P.H., R.D., author of *Why Women Need Chocolate*. (See Habit 1: Mindless Eating for more on breakfast and mood.)

Regular exercise, a strong social support system, adequate sleep, and limited alcohol consumption are other reinforcements for contending with a grumpy mood or low energy. But dietwise, it's the carbs, caffeine, and sugar in the foods you eat—and when you eat them—that have the most profound effect on how raring to go you are after lunch, whether you snap at a coworker, and how often you forget where you put your keys. What you ate earlier in the day could even play a role in whether you dive into the chocolate after work. Instead of turning to doughnuts and Doritos when you're anxious, crabby, or tired, follow a few simple, smart guidelines and you'll not only eat healthier but feel better, too.

Food and Mood

It's no coincidence that we seize on carbohydrate-rich foods such as pasta or pie when we feel stressed, tired, or blue. "People unconsciously self-medicate by turning to sweets or other carb-heavy snacks in an effort to feel better," says Waterhouse. Carbs raise levels of serotonin, a neurotransmitter in the brain that elevates mood and suppresses appetite. In contrast, low-carb/high-protein diets reduce serotonin levels, which explains why some people report feeling fatigued or down in the dumps when they follow these weight-loss plans. Several conditions associated with moodiness and fatigue—from premenstrual syndrome to winter blues—are linked to low serotonin levels and increased cravings for carb-rich foods, such as candy, cookies, cakes, and other desserts. Serotonin levels are partially regulated by sunlight: the higher the exposure, the more serotonin that's produced in the brain. "Our exposure to sunlight, however, drops during winter, which helps to explain why some women feel more fatigued and stressed and have stronger PMS and menopausal symptoms this time of year," says Waterhouse.

When you eat carbs, however, is key. That's because besides boosting mood, serotonin also relaxes you. A study from Kansas State University found that women who drank sugary (i.e., carb-loaded) beverages were sleepier within a half hour of consumption compared with women who drank water or diet drinks. So, chowing down on a carb-packed meal could dull your concentration and leave you feeling groggy, which may be fine in the evening after dinner but could interfere with a board meeting in midafternoon.

Your crave control is a product of more than just serotonin. A preference for toast, waffles, or pancakes at breakfast could be triggered by the nerve chemical neuropeptide Y (NPY), which encourages us to restock glucose stores, while a hankering for meat, ice cream, salad with dressing, or other fatty foods could be triggered by different nerve chemicals, including galanin or the endorphins. Regardless, the solution is simple: work with your cravings, rather than against them. "Ignore these messages, and the pendulum might swing from abstinence to binge, especially on those days when your emotions are in full force," says Waterhouse.

Coffee and Your Jitter Threshold

The promise of instant energy has made caffeine the number one mind-altering drug. The caffeine in coffee, tea, and cola blocks a nerve chemical called adenosine that calms us down. As a result, we are more alert, react faster, and concentrate better within half an hour of drinking a cup of java or downing a cola.

Unfortunately, caffeine is a double-edged sword. Drinking too much fuels fatigue, which is one of the first symptoms of caffeine withdrawal. It also can make you too jittery to concentrate or cause you to feel a bit blue. Studies published in *Behavior Therapy* and the *Journal of Abnormal Psychology* found that removing caffeine (or sugar) from the diets of people battling depression

Foods to Boost Mood

Omega-3 Fats

Benefits: Cultures in which people consume ample amounts of omega-3 fats have up to a sixtyfold lower incidence of depression, compared with cultures in which people include little or none of the omega-3s. Studies in which people have been given omega-3-rich fish oil capsules or placebos have shown lowered levels of depression. "We see up to a 50 percent reduction in depression in people who are the toughest to treat, such as people who are unresponsive to medication. But you don't have to be clinically depressed to benefit from the omega-3 fats, since including these fats in the diet improves feelings of well-being even in people who just battle common, everyday blues," says Joseph Hibbeln, M.D., who has specialized in omega-3 research. Low blood and tissue levels of omega-3s also are markers for inadequate serotonin, which is strongly associated with depression. The omega-3s also might help people cope with stress.

Foods to Eat: Seafood, especially fatty fish such as salmon, herring, and mackerel; walnuts; flaxseed meal; rapeseed oil.

Folic Acid

Benefits: This B vitamin helps nerve cells manufacture several of the neurotransmitters that regulate mood and mind. It also lowers levels of a brain- and artery-damaging substance called homocysteine. So, it's no surprise that poor intake is often linked with depression and memory loss, while optimal intake improves mood, attention, and mental function.

Foods to Eat: Dark green leafies, such as spinach, chard, kale, and romaine; legumes; oranges; peanuts. Small amounts are found in sunflower seeds, whole grains, and fortified refined grains.

Antioxidants

Benefits: The body depends on antioxidants—from vitamins C and E to thousands of phytochemicals—to protect against cell damage and memory loss caused by free radicals, which are highly reactive oxygen fragments generated by stress hormones.

Foods to Eat: Rich-colored fruits and vegetables, such as dried plums, berries, sweet potatoes, carrots, broccoli, tomatoes, purple grapes, and mangoes; green tea; whole grains.

improved mood and energy level within two weeks. "A common finding was that these people first reported they had more energy, and then their depression improved," says study author Larry Christensen, Ph.D., now department chair in psychology at the University of South Alabama.

Sugar Rush

We are eating more sugar than ever—up to 31 teaspoons of added sugar a day, according to the latest stats from the U.S. Department of Agriculture (USDA). All that sweetness could undermine our moods. When we eat sweets, sugar is dumped into the bloodstream, prompting a temporary blood sugar spike that's followed by a sudden drop—usually to levels lower than they were *before* the sugary snack. This can leave you feeling irritable, tired, depressed, or jittery. As with caffeine, using sugar to self-regulate your mood is a temporary fix. "People who turn to sweets or coffee may relieve fatigue and feel better temporarily, but the symptoms return," says Christensen. The person then reaches for another sugar fix, and a vicious cycle develops. Eliminating sugar or caffeine from the diet can be a permanent solution for many people battling depression, according to Christensen. Cutting back is a good idea for everyone.

There's an obvious reason why we turn to all the wrong comforting sweet foods—such as chocolate chip cookies, milkshakes, and cheeseburgers and fries—during times of stress. These foods blunt the stress response and calm us down, according to research conducted at the University of California, San Francisco. The stress hormones apparently prompt the typical fight-or-flight response as well as signal the brain to seek foods high in sugar and fat, which in turn dampen the stress response and help us cope. In essence, sweet and creamy foods provide a brake on the brain's chronic stress response. In the studies, animals exposed to stress showed a marked reduction in their reaction to stress when fed high-calorie, sweet-and-fatty foods. Mary Dallman, Ph.D., head researcher on the study, believes that the animals are a good model for how humans respond to eating and stress. A study from Pennsylvania State University supports this connection and found that women who feel overwhelmed by stress eat twice the amount of fatty snacks as do stress-resistant women, even after the stress is over.

This makes sense from an evolutionary standpoint, in that the body needs calories to fight off or escape a threat—such as a saber-toothed tiger in days gone by. Once the energy stores are replenished, the body will signal an end to this craving. But in our modern-day world, free of saber-toothed tigers, day-in-and-day-out chronic stress keeps the "eat now" signal jammed. Sally, a graphic artist in Bend, Oregon, says she knows all too well how low-grade chronic stress can cause you to eat: "I am rarely physically hungry. Instead, I just eat all day long, mostly out of nerves and the demands of my job. I sit at a computer, trying to be creative. Constant snacking has become both a distraction and a way to soothe myself and stay focused." Stay-at-home moms also can easily succumb to a food craving when the kids get on their nerves. Victoria, a freelance writer in Portland, Oregon, admits: "Being at home with a two- and four-year-old all day can be trying and tiring. I find the afternoons to be particularly difficult, especially if I know that my husband is working late and I have several more hours to go before I have any relief from the nonstop kid demands. Sweets and chocolate become my comfort and reward; they keep my spirits up and get me through the late afternoon."

The downside is that the stress hormones also activate fat receptors in the abdomen, forcing any extra calories into fat storage, otherwise known as your love handles, saddlebags, belly, hips, and thighs. "Chronic stress jams the stress hormone cortisol into high gear, which increases cravings for foods rich in carbohydrates and fat and encourages any excess calories to be stored in the belly, where they are readily available to fuel the stress response," explains Pamela Peeke, M.D., assistant clinical professor of medicine at the University of Maryland School of Medicine and author of *Body for Life for Women*. It follows that stressed-out people who overeat in response to emotions also gain more fat around the middle, a type of weight gain associated with elevated risks for heart disease, diabetes, hypertension, and cancer.

Sugar Addiction

Turning to sugar once in a while to calm frazzled nerves probably won't hurt, but repeated trips to the cookie jar could lead to weight gain and could even be addicting. Many women have known all along that sweets are addicting, but for years, experts speculated that sugar addiction was an issue of habit, not substance abuse. Recent research at Princeton University changed all that. "We found in our studies that animals fed high-sugar diets exhibit all the symptoms of withdrawal, including agitation and nervousness, when sugar is taken away," says Bartley Hoebel, Ph.D., professor of psychology at Princeton. "Reintroduce sugar to their diets and the animals binge, all of which are classic symptoms of substance abuse."

Changes in the animals' brains also resemble changes seen in morphine and heroin addiction. The very taste of sugar on the tongue releases endorphins, neurotransmitters that act much like morphine to provide a pleasurable response. Another neurotransmitter, dopamine, permanently stamps the experience into our memory banks so that we are programmed to seek this yummy taste again. We literally become dependent on an inborn "high," feeling both comforted and pleasured whenever we eat sugar. The response is so powerful that even the sight of food, let alone the smell, at a later date releases dopamine and a craving for another sweet taste and mood fix.

Sugar addiction is by no means as powerful or harmful as a drug addiction, but this research should be comforting to all those women who have been undone by a sweet tooth. Don't scold yourself. Craving a cookie is not a willpower problem or a sign that you're a bad person. You really might be hooked on sugar!

Dieting = Weight Gain

Women who diet are especially prone to overeating when they get grumpy, feel stressed, or are premenstrual. Severe dieting numbs the hunger response, so women lose the ability to know when they're hungry or full. Instead, they are likely to interpret any emotional discomfort and all troubling feelings as hunger.

It's an understandable trade-off. Probably nothing else in life is as firmly rooted in security as is food. "As babies, the most powerful comforter when we are distressed is food, so it makes sense that we would continue to turn to that symbol of comfort as adults. Grabbing a cookie is like trying to return to that security, that home, that safe place," says Carol Munter, coauthor of *When Women Stop Hating Their Bodies*. Thus, food becomes a tranquilizer when we're anxious and a mood elevator when we're depressed. It fills us up when we're emotionally starved, comforts us when we're lonely, and entertains us when we're bored. Unfortunately, turning to food for something other than physical nourishment only trades one problem for another.

Are You Overeating?

Women sometimes think they are overeating, when in fact they're not eating enough. The Food and Nutrition Board (the same group that developed the Recommended Dietary Allowances) recommends that a moderately active woman who is 5'5" tall and weighs 128 to 138 pounds should consume about 2,200 calories daily. If you're eating fewer than 1,600 to 2,000 calories daily (depending on your height, age, and activity level), then you're undereating, not overeating. But, how do you know if you're eating too much or not enough? What does a real meal look like?

The basic day's menu should include at least 6 grains (at least 3 whole grains), 5 (preferably 8 to 10) fruits and vegetables, 3 calcium-rich selections such as nonfat milk or yogurt, and 2–3 iron-rich selections such as extra-lean meat, chicken, fish, or legumes. You should eat regularly throughout the day, or at least five times, so every minimeal or snack should include at least 1 grain and 1 to 2 fruits or vegetables. At three of those meals or snacks, you also should include a calcium-rich and an iron-rich selection. All in all, about three-quarters of your plate will be grains, produce, and legumes, with the remainder being meat and/or milk products.

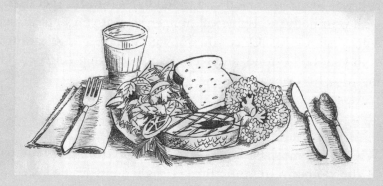

For any woman who has lost the sense of true hunger, it's a slow road back to getting in touch with her body, hunger, and physical needs, but the rewards are worth it. Munter says that women who give up the diet mentality and relearn how to nurture themselves experience a new lease on life.

Kick the Habit

Some women know that they eat for emotional reasons and are ready to kick the habit. Other women might not even know this is a problem; they have been eating in response to mood rather than hunger for so long that they don't recognize the difference.

That's where record keeping comes into play, as explained in Habit 1: Mindless Eating. Keep a food journal for a week, writing down everything you eat and how much. This time, though, add a third category: how do you feel before and after eating? Ask yourself, before you wolf down that meal, how you feel. Are you relaxed, anxious, sad, lonely, stressed, happy, excited, depressed, bored? Also check in with your body and write down, on a scale of 1 to 5, how physically hungry you are. After you've eaten, again record how you feel—satisfied, full, relaxed, anxious, happy, bored, and so forth. At the end of the week, compare the before and after feelings to identify whether emotions or true hunger pangs are triggering you to eat. Use the "Food and Mood Journal" (next page) as a template for keeping these records.

If you know that emotions enter in to your food choices, the best way to kick the food and mood habit is to first get in touch with your body's real physical hunger, so that you stop eating for emotional reasons. Once you do, your next goal is to eat in tune with your body, mind, and feelings rather than giving in to cravings that lead you astray.

Get in Touch with Hunger

What does physical hunger feel like? It is growling or mild pangs in the stomach, or sometimes a slight light-headed feeling as blood sugar begins to drop. Your goal is to eat regularly throughout the day, and usually only when you're physically hungry.

Food and Mood Journal

For one week, write down everything you eat and how much, as well as your mood both before and after eating. Prior to each meal or snack, rate your physical hunger level from 1 to 5 (1 = not hungry at all, 5 = ravenous). Review your records to identify whether you eat for real hunger or in response to emotions. Also look for patterns, such as the types of foods you choose in response to different emotions. Make copies of this form, or use it as an example to develop your own journal.

Date: _____

Time of Day	Food Chosen	Amount	Hunger (1–5)	Thoughts/Feelings Before	After
____	____	____	____	____	____
____	____	____	____	____	____
____	____	____	____	____	____
____	____	____	____	____	____
____	____	____	____	____	____
____	____	____	____	____	____
____	____	____	____	____	____
____	____	____	____	____	____

The most important solution for emotional eating is to find comfort somewhere other than food. Thomas Wadden, Ph.D., professor of psychology and director of the Weight and Eating Disorders Program at the University of Pennsylvania, recommends, "Talk through, rather than eat through, those feelings." Mary Dallman agrees and notes that nipping stress in the bud can help inhibit the stress response that otherwise leads to overindulging in high-calorie comfort foods. She advises, "Read a book, walk in the woods, or go for a bike ride on a regular basis as preventive measures before you are so tense that you overeat and pack on the pounds." John Foreyt adds: "Any change is stressful, even changing to a healthier eating style. So, before you take the plunge into any new eating program, take stock of your feelings and pay attention to any potential sources of increased stress or anxiety."

Learn to identify your feelings and fulfill the associated needs by means other than food, such as exercising daily, spending time in nature, developing close friendships, meditating, or even talking to a counselor. Valerie, an airport security manager in Portland, Oregon, attests: "I used to eat when I was having a bad day, but now I do yard work, play with my birds, call a friend, or work out. After any of those stress-busters, it's hard to be anything but tired, relaxed, or downright happy." She adds that when she is stressed, she gathers a gossip magazine, some candles, and a glass of wine and heads for a good, long soak in a bubble bath.

Here are other habits to adopt when you need to keep emotional eating at bay:

- **Listen to your body.** Tune in to your natural hunger signals, making a distinction between what Munter calls "mouth hunger" (psychological hunger) and "stomach hunger" (true hunger—symptoms include an emptiness in your stomach and stomach rumblings). If you are truly hungry, don't deny yourself. Ask yourself, "What would satisfy this particular hunger?" Then eat what seems like a good match.
- **Eat mindfully.** Pay attention to and enjoy every mouthful. Halfway through a meal, stop, sit back, and pay attention to

your body. If you still feel physically hungry, then have another few bites, stop, and listen again. Stop for good when you are comfortably full.

- **Graze—don't gorge.** "Start feeding yourself on demand, as you would feed a baby," Munter recommends. By reparenting ourselves, we learn to trust that food will always be there, and we begin to feel more secure in general. Eat minimeals every four hours or whenever you are physically hungry. Choose real foods, such as baby carrots, blueberries, yogurt, half of a whole-wheat bagel, or a handful of nuts.

- **Be patient with yourself.** Until you have reprogrammed your attitudes toward food and no longer feel deprived, there's always the chance you'll overeat when feeling moody. Your goal is to gradually lean in the direction of eating for physical hunger and away from emotional hunger.

- **Focus on health, not weight.** "Women who have dieted all their lives are often afraid to give up the diet mentality and eat at will; they're afraid they'll gain an enormous amount of weight," says Munter. In reality, your weight will stabilize when you "legalize food," and even if you gain a few pounds in the beginning, over time you will return to what for you is a normal, healthy weight. Some women do gain a little weight, but most lose some or stay the same; most important is that when women are released from the 24-hour-a-day pressure of food obsession, they say, "What a relief to finally be myself!"

Fuel a Good Mood

The whole subject of dealing with out-of-whack appetites and grumpy moods might come down to focusing on real, unprocessed foods and your health. "The critical issue is that it is fat, sugar, and salt we overeat when we are feeling blue; you never hear anyone say, 'I just can't stop eating celery,'" says Adam Drewnowski, Ph.D., of the University of Washington.

Carbs have been getting a bad rap lately, including blame for obesity and heart disease. Yet, these very carbs have the power to

Healthy Munchies to Soothe Your Mood

Here are 25 snacks that require about the same amount of time to fix that it takes to grab a diet cola and a bag of chips, but that also calm your nerves and soothe your moods while fueling your body. Most are portable, so remember to take some along when you leave the house! As always, watch portion sizes: even if a snack is healthful, eating two or three times too much can add hundreds of calories to your diet and inches to your hips.

1. 1 cup of low-fat vanilla yogurt mixed with 1 tablespoon of slivered almonds and 1 tablespoon of raisins. Serve with a banana and bottled water.
2. Two fig bars and 1 cup of low-fat milk.
3. Half a cantaloupe filled with 6 ounces of low-fat lemon yogurt (optional: 1 teaspoon of lemon zest).
4. ½ cup of all-fruit sorbet, ½ cup of fresh berries, and bottled water.
5. ⅔ cup of grapes, three graham crackers, and 1 cup of light vanilla soy milk.
6. Convenience store snack: a 6-ounce container of low-fat yogurt, a small pouch of trail mix, a banana, and bottled water.
7. 1 ounce of extra-lean sandwich ham cut into strips and placed on top of six low-fat whole-wheat crackers. Serve with an apple and bottled water.
8. 1 cup of 1 percent low-fat milk, warmed and flavored with almond extract. Serve with a banana and 1 ounce of peanuts.
9. A thin slice of date-nut bread topped with fat-free cream cheese and three pitted dates. Serve with a glass of 1 percent low-fat milk or light soy milk.
10. A large apple, quartered and seeded and drizzled with 1 teaspoon of caramel sauce. Serve with ½ cup of low-fat cottage cheese.

11. Ten cherry tomatoes hollowed out and filled with left-over tuna salad, hummus, or couscous. Serve with sparkling water.
12. Ten slices of cucumber topped with fat-free cream cheese, leftover cooked shrimp, and commercial cocktail sauce.
13. Baked tortilla chips dipped in fat-free refried beans and commercial salsa. Serve with orange juice mixed with sparkling water. (Two great premade bean dips are Trader Joe's Smoky Black Bean Dip and Salpica Chipotle Black Bean Dip.)
14. Homemade snack mix: no-salt whole-wheat pretzels, dried fruit, and toasted almonds.
15. StarKist "Lunch to Go" snack pack—chunk light tuna, low-calorie mayo, pickle relish, and six crackers. Serve with an orange.
16. ¼ cup of soy nuts (Mighty Mo Munches is especially good) and canned fruit, drained.
17. Apple sandwiches made by spreading nut butter between thin slices of apple. Serve with a glass of soy milk.
18. Twenty fresh cherries, 1 ounce of almonds, and a glass of low-fat milk.
19. A bowl of canned low-sodium bean soup, a slice of whole-wheat bread, and orange slices.
20. Chickpeas rinsed and drained and sprinkled with garlic powder, paprika, and lemon. Serve with grapefruit juice.
21. A sliced whole-wheat bagel topped with fat-free cream cheese, a romaine leaf, and a tomato slice.
22. Leftover chicken, fish, or beans wrapped in a large leaf of romaine.
23. A banana, a handful of strawberries, and soy milk or yogurt whipped in a blender.
24. Leftover rice topped with ½ cup of canned black beans.
25. A leftover baked sweet potato sliced and drizzled with maple syrup and chopped walnuts.

Quality Carbs

Quality carbs come from fruits, vegetables, legumes (black beans, kidney beans, garbanzos, lentils, split peas, etc.), and whole grains. All "soothe" your brain chemistry, while fueling your body, health, and longevity. Most whole grains can be found at your local supermarket or health food store.

Grain Varieties	How to Use
Wheat	
Whole-wheat flour	Any way you use flour
Bulgur or cracked wheat	As pilaf, stuffings, breakfast cereal
Wheat berries	As pilaf, stuffings, breakfast cereal
Wheat bran	Add to baked goods and cereal
Whole-wheat couscous	Any way you use rice
Wheat germ	Add to baked goods, pancakes, waffles, bread dough, meat loaf, meatballs; sprinkle on cereal
Barley	
Pearled	Add to soups, risotto, salads; any way you use rice
Brown Rice	
Brown rice flour	In baked goods and noodles
Other forms	In side dishes, rice pudding, stuffings, stir-fries, rice and bean salads, soups; as a base for creamed dishes; cooked cereal
Buckwheat	
Flour	Pancakes, blini

| Roasted buckwheat groats (kasha) | In place of rice where earthy flavor will not overwhelm other ingredients |

Oats
Rolled or steel-cut — Cooked cereal, baked goods

(You can purchase most of the following lesser-known whole grains at your local health food store, through mail order, or from websites.)

Quinoa
(Small, round, ivory-colored grain; high in protein; mild-tasting; quick-cooking) — In side dishes, stuffed bell peppers, chowders, bean/grain salads

Amaranth
(Tiny, mustard-colored seed; nutty, peppery flavor; also available as flour) — Mix with other grains for a side dish

Wild Rice
(Chewy texture, earthy flavor) — In side dishes and stuffings; mix with brown rice in pilafs, salads, and as complement to main course

Spelt
(An ancient form of wheat; low in gluten) — Use as wheat; good for people with gluten intolerance

Wehani Rice
(Mahogany-colored whole grain; robust, nutty flavor and chewy texture) — Use as rice

improve our moods and pull us out of a funk. The problem with carbs is that we are eating too much of the wrong stuff, serving up platters of pasta, softball-size muffins, and other refined grains high in sugar, refined flour, and fat. According to the USDA, Americans today average 300 more daily calories than in 1985, and almost half of those extra calories come from refined and processed carbs.

Downing excessive amounts of refined grains and sugary foods can definitely add inches to your waistline, but replacing at least half the refined grains in your diet with fiber-rich whole grains helps raise serotonin levels and enhance mood, while keeping you trim. According to researchers at Tufts University, people who load up on fiber-rich foods, such as whole grains, feel satisfied and less hungry than do people who chow down on processed grains. Adding as little as 14 grams of extra whole-grain fiber to your diet lowers your calorie intake by about 10 percent, which could result in up to a 4-pound drop in weight. It's as easy as eating a bowl of whole-grain cereal for breakfast, a turkey sandwich on whole-wheat bread at lunch, and a side of instant brown rice at dinner.

Combine quality carbs with protein at every meal to fuel your body, mind, and mood, while curbing swells in blood sugar. This is as easy as having oatmeal (grain) with low-fat milk (protein) and fruit for breakfast, turkey breast (protein) on whole-wheat bread (grain) with a salad for lunch, and grilled salmon (protein) with brown rice (grain) and vegetables at dinner. Midafternoon can be the high point of the day for carb cravings, so plan ahead and have a nutritious all-carb snack, such as a bowl of air-popped popcorn, a toasted whole-grain English muffin with jam, or half a cinnamon-raisin bagel with honey and fruit. In addition, follow these simple steps:

- **Take it slowly.** Attempting any dietary change too rapidly can throw these appetite-control chemicals into chaos. A gradual change in eating habits is more effective: you work *with* your brain's chemistry, rather than against it.

- **Don't ignore your neurotransmitters.** Skipping breakfast causes NPY levels to escalate, contributing to overeating later in the day. Allowing more than four to five hours to go by between meals causes the release of fat fragments from fat tissue, which will amplify appetite to a full-scale binge. "If someone reports struggling with food cravings in the afternoon, my first question is, 'Did you eat breakfast?' More often than not, the answer is no," says C. Wayne Callaway, M.D., of George Washington University. He recommends eating regularly throughout the day, which, over the course of a few weeks, will help reprogram the body's appetite and hunger clock.
- **Choose foods that satisfy.** Adorn your plate with vegetables, fruits, whole grains, and legumes, which fill you up without filling you out. Include a little protein in each meal and snack, since both protein and complex carbs increase satiation, so you eat less and feel full longer.
- **Focus on flavor.** Add canned chilies or roasted red peppers to a chicken sandwich, salsa to scrambled eggs, and nutmeg to peaches, and you'll satisfy your senses, without overeating.
- **Cut down on fat.** Fat has a low satiety quotient, so it takes more food to fill us up, resulting in passive overconsumption of calories. All animals studied, from rats and mice to dogs and humans, overeat and gain weight when fed high-fat diets. The high-fat meals also increase both the size and number of fat cells, making it increasingly difficult to lose the weight later on.
- **Take a multivitamin and mineral supplement to fill in the gaps on days when you don't eat perfectly.** Vitamins and minerals, such as vitamins B_{12} and B_6, folic acid, and iron, are important assembly-line workers that help the body make neurotransmitters, carry oxygen to the brain, and maintain healthy, functioning nerves, which influence your mood and level of energy.
- **Drink water.** Even mild dehydration can lead to headaches and fatigue. The recommended daily intake is 11 cups for

women. Food supplies about 20 percent of that, so make up the difference by aiming for at least eight glasses of liquid every day, including water, tea, coffee, juices, and other beverages.

If you battle depression, try eliminating sugar from your diet. For everyone else, going easy on sugar is a good idea, too. Experts recommend that we limit intake of added sugars to 12 teaspoons a day, which means trimming our typical intake by two-thirds. To do that, read labels, and limit foods that list sugar or any of its aliases (such as high-fructose corn syrup, glucose, sucrose, or

The Six Food Rules to Manage Your Mood

Rule 1: Make sure every meal contains foods rich in complex carbohydrates. Also, plan a carbohydrate-rich snack, such as whole-grain crackers and peanut butter, an onion bagel with low-fat cheese, or baked tortilla chips and low-fat bean dip, to curb midafternoon snack attacks.

Rule 2: Cut back on sugar-containing foods, including desserts, sugarcoated cereals, candy, sugar-sweetened beverages, and sugary snack foods such as granola bars. Manage sweet cravings by replacing refined sweets with nutrient-packed foods, such as fresh fruit, crunchy vegetables, whole-grain bagels, or low-fat yogurt.

Rule 3: Cut back on caffeine from coffee, tea, chocolate, cocoa, colas, and medications. Drink more water instead.

Rule 4: Increase dietary intake of vitamin B_6—a nutrient that helps boost serotonin levels—by including several servings daily of foods such as chicken, legumes, fish, bananas, avocados, and dark green leafy vegetables. Whole grains are preferable to refined, enriched grains, since more than

70 percent of the vitamin is lost during processing. Also, include at least two foods that are rich in folic acid in your daily diet, such as spinach, broccoli, orange juice, and chard.

Rule 5: Make changes gradually. Select two or three small changes, and practice these until they are comfortable. Then select two more. This will help assure long-term success in sticking with your plan and will allow your brain chemistry time to adjust to the new eating style without throwing your nerve chemicals into a tailspin.

Rule 6: Take a moderate-dose multiple vitamin and mineral supplement to fill in any nutritional gaps.

honey) among the first three ingredients or that list several sugars throughout the ingredient list. Cut soft drinks to one a week, since these are the principal source of sugar in many people's diets. You still can have your favorite treats; just limit the portion to an occasional cookie or small slice of cake. Moderation, after all, is key to a healthful diet. Finally, have your sweet treat at the end of a meal, to avoid the blood sugar roller-coaster ride that comes when you eat sweets alone.

Curb the caffeine fix. If you are grumpy but not necessarily clinically depressed, then there is no need to give up coffee. A cup or two a day is probably safe (unless you are supersensitive to caffeine, in which case, avoid caffeine altogether for two weeks and see if you notice an improvement in sleep, mood, and energy level). However, if you drink coffee, tea, or cola all day long, you might want to throttle back. Sidestep caffeine-withdrawal headaches by switching to half caffeinated and half decaffeinated beverages, and slowly reduce the number of servings during a two-week weaning period. Limit your caffeine to morning and early afternoon, since caffeine can linger in the body for hours, interfering with a good night's sleep.

Looking for an alternative to coffee to boost your energy? Try eating regularly. Divide food intake into five or more little meals and snacks evenly dispersed throughout the day. "Your thinking, energy, and mood will suffer if you skip breakfast and have a big lunch. Eating a light snack or meal every four hours that combines a mix of protein and quality carbs improves mental alertness and work performance," says Susan Moores, M.S., R.D., spokesperson for the American Dietetic Association.

Your Mood Is More than Just Diet

Breaking the habit of eating to soothe emotions is only part of escaping the mood muddle. Regular exercise, effective coping skills, a strong social support system, and limiting or avoiding alcohol, cigarettes, and medications that compound an emotional problem also are important considerations. Depression also can be a symptom of other problems, so always consult a physician if emotional problems persist or interfere long term with the quality of your life and health. In the meantime, keep in mind that what you choose to soothe your hunger also will be fueling your mood.

Give Me the Quick Fix, Now!

If it hadn't been on one of the top morning shows that I heard it, I might have ignored the statement. But, there it was as large as life: another celebrity diet-guru touting an age-old myth that eating the wrong combination of foods—in this case, fat and sugar at the same meal—leads to a metabolism meltdown and ultimately weight gain. Avoid this food combination, and the weight just melts right off—no effort, no other change in eating habits, no exercise, no hunger, no problem. Thus we arrive at Habit 8.

Popular beliefs about dieting come and go, but the message is the same; just the face and the pitch change. Kelly Brownell, Ph.D., professor of psychology at Yale and a pioneer in weight-management research, warns, "Since the government doesn't regulate diet claims, people make outlandish statements and can sell or say anything when it comes to weight loss."

We might have been hook, line, and sinkered in the past by fat-burning creams, liquid protein drinks, cider vinegar and kelp diets, starch blockers, aromatherapy, acupressure, herbs that melt cellulite, and pills that metabolize fat, but aren't we more skeptical of diet claims these days? Not according to Brownell: "When people look for that edge, an advantage for weight loss, it's easy to miss the forest for the trees." Welcome to one of the most powerful habits that mess up women's diets: falling for the latest fad gimmick.

We are obsessed with a desire to be thin. More than 70 million Americans and more than 4 in every 10 women are dieting right now, cutting carbs, taking weight-loss supplements, joining diet groups, slurping canned milkshake-like diet drinks, and spending almost $50 billion annually on one diet aid after another. Most of those dieters have heard the warning that diets don't work. Still, they fall for scam after scam.

How to Spot a Gimmick

Here are 10 warnings signs of a fad diet.

1. Recommendations that promise a quick, effortless fix.
2. Claims that sound too good to be true, such as that you'll lose more than 2 pounds a week, weight loss is effortless, or you can eat all you want.
3. Restriction or elimination of healthy foods; recommendations of certain food combinations or large amounts of some foods; and rigid, inflexible eating plans.
4. Recommendations based on a single study or on overly simplified conclusions drawn from a complex study.
5. Dramatic statements that are refuted by reputable scientific studies or organizations.
6. Lists of "good" and "bad" foods, or promotion of miracle foods, herbs, or nutrients.
7. Recommendations made to help sell a product.
8. Recommendations based on studies published without peer review or based on testimonials, anecdotes, and stories.
9. Recommendations from studies that ignore differences among individuals or groups.
10. Statements that weight can be lost and that the loss can be maintained with little or no exercise or other changes in lifestyle.

Diets really don't work. Really. Oh sure, you'll lose a few pounds in the beginning on a low-carb diet, an all-soup diet, or a food-combining diet. You'll initially drop some weight eating according to your blood type, body type, personality type, or metabolic type. You might even lose a pound or two taking the latest diet pill—these days it's propolene, bovine collagen, and green tea capsules. That's because you've cut calories. You lose weight on any diet, from a sugar-free to an all-sugar diet, when you reduce calories. Few, if any, of these kamikaze diets teach us how to eat right, and none of them help us maintain the weight we might initially lose. Instead, we eliminate foods, restrict calories, skip meals, and essentially abuse our bodies in a desperate effort to drop a dress size. Most of these diets are time-consuming, annoying, and woefully unsatisfying. Once the novelty wears off, so does the motivation to keep at it. Up to 80 percent of us gain back the weight and more, finding we sacrificed our health and have learned zilch about what it takes to be healthy and fit.

The news is not all gloomy. One in five women *does* lose weight and keep the weight off. We know exactly how they do it: They get real. They get committed. They get determined. Regardless of their dieting history, this time something clicked, and the success stories say, on reflecting back, that they were relentless in their decision to make this the last—and successful—diet. They stopped the quick-fix approach and developed plans they would live with for the rest of their lives.

Dieting can work, even when fad diets don't. Let's take a look at why fads always fail us, and then explore how you can kick the fad-diet habit, successfully lose weight, and, more important, keep the weight off!

Tell Me Again Why Diets Don't Work

Most fad diets work pretty well for a while. It's the long-term results where they fail miserably, with more than 9 out of 10 fad dieters gaining the weight back, and then gaining even more—even worse statistics than those for the more common nonfad diets. Fad diets might get you into that slinky dress for your class reunion or a sister's wedding, but rarely do they get you in shape for the rest of your life.

One reason for the high failure rate of fad diets is that the diets are based on deprivation. Take away a woman's freedom to choose, and she begins to crave the very thing she can't have. "The more food is off limits, and the more we worry about what we're eating, count calories and fat grams, and lament our lack of willpower, the more we eat," says Carol Munter, coauthor of *Overcoming Overeating.* "The end result of dieting," she emphasizes, "is compulsive overeating." Research at the University of Toronto supports this thesis, finding that women become food-obsessed when dieting. All they talk about is food, recipes, and restaurants. Boring! This single-mindedness leads them to overeat. The best that can happen from dieting is that we overeat once in a while. At worst, we develop severe eating disorders such as binge eating or bulimia.

The link between dieting and food obsession is nothing new. During World War II, Dr. Ancel Keys, a University of Minnesota public-health professor who invented the K-ration, studied the effects of food restriction on a group of conscientious objectors who cut calories by 25 percent for six months. As they lost weight, their interest in food intensified. They talked about food; they fantasized about food; they collected recipes; they developed bizarre eating rituals. Sound like someone you know on a diet? Today's dieters are under even more pressure; unlike the conscientious objectors, they are constantly exposed to food and dieting messages from the media, society, and friends. It's no wonder they develop the habit of eating more than their nondieting friends whenever they try to eat less.

As illustrated in the preceding chapter, dieters lose the ability to recognize real hunger messages from their bodies. They ignore their feelings of hunger and fullness and, instead, adjust to the habit of eating based on the rules of the diet. Without those valuable internal messages, your mind takes over and makes up all kinds of excuses for why it's OK to eat: "I exercised today, so I can have a piece of cheesecake," "I had low-fat yogurt for lunch, so I can have a second piece of pie tonight," "If I skip lunch, I can have twice as much for dinner," "I didn't have my regular bag of chips yesterday, so today I can have two bags," and so forth. They also mistake emotional discomfort for physical hunger, so they're more prone to emotional eating, mindless eating, and rationalizing their poor food choices.

A dieter's body loses control over eating as the diet takes over. Diets are not strong taskmasters, so the first time a woman feels irritable, tired, or angry and comes upon a box of chocolates, she throws in the towel. In another study from the University of Toronto, dieting and nondieting women were first given milkshakes to drink and then asked to taste-test three samples of ice creams. The nondieters consumed a little bit of each sample, but the dieters, having dropped their guard with the milkshake, binged on the ice cream—gobbling pints, not spoonfuls. Other studies show that women eat more just anticipating going on a diet!

This seesaw of abstaining and gorging is often what leads women from one fad diet to the next. One women comments, "I followed the *Fit for Life* diet and lost about 60 pounds, but the abstinence did me in. I am a big breakfast eater, and once I went back to that, I went back to all the old habits and gained more than twice as much weight as I'd lost. It wasn't until I found an eating style where I didn't deny myself anything, but stayed on top of calories and portions, that I finally lost the weight for good."

Another problem with fad diets is that they don't teach you how to eat sensibly. You gain the weight back when you go "off the diet" and return to your old eating ways. "It's much harder to maintain weight loss if a woman lost the weight on a fad diet, probably because she didn't develop the habits along the way to sustain her when the diet was over," says Fletcher.

Worse yet, no get-thin-quick diet supplies optimal levels of all the nutrients your body needs to be healthy. Whether it's the Beverly Hills Diet, the California Diet, the Rotation Diet, the F-Plan Diet, the Carbohydrate Addict's Diet, the Cortisol Diet, the Goddess Diet, the Warrior Diet, the Zone Diet, the Never-Say-Diet Diet, the Martini Diet, the Coconut Diet, the Grapefruit Diet, or the Stillman, Atkins, New Atkins, Scarsdale, Rosedale, or Schwarzbein diet, every fad diet analyzed was shown to be low in some to all nutrients studied. Some are high in harmful substances, such as saturated fat and cholesterol. Others ban foods known to help lower disease risk, such as watermelon and carrots. Few people maintain any weight loss; they seriously jeopardize their health for their waistlines, all for nothing.

Diet Myths Debunked

Most of us would pay any price for the diet trick that would really and truly take off the pounds forever. In the mad scramble for the latest diet secret, we blindly launch into food combining, carb bashing, or munching on diet bars, while overlooking or underrating the best habits of all—the ones that successful dieters swear by, the ones that have proved their worth over decades. "The tried-and-true secret to losing weight, whether it is on a diet or because of sensible lifestyle changes, is that you must cut calories, increase physical activity, or both," says Brownell. Here's the scoop on some of the most popular, but overrated, trends and, more important, how to use some of the best, yet underrated, diet habits to maximize your weight-loss success.

Food Combining

Despite the claims made by that celebrity diet-guru, there is no evidence that weight problems develop because we eat foods in the wrong combination, such as mixing sugar with fat at a meal, according to John Foreyt, Ph.D., director of the Nutrition Research Center at Baylor College of Medicine. Our bodies were designed over hundreds of thousands of years to readily digest and thrive on a wide variety of foods and food mixtures. Beliefs that protein and carb or fat and carb don't mix go against both common sense and everything known about digestion. Besides, almost all foods (except sugar, oils, and most fruits) are already a combination of carbs, protein, and fat. (A slice of any type of bread contains 3 grams of protein, 16 grams of carbs, and 1½ grams of fat; a bowl of black beans is a nice combo of 15 grams of protein, 41 grams of carbs, and 1 gram of fat; and even broccoli contains a little bit of all three nutrients.) "This diet fad is a complete hoax," Foreyt concludes.

On the other hand, a balanced mix of high-quality carbs (whole grains and starchy vegetables) and protein with a small amount of fat is what counts for weight loss. Protein and carbs are more satiating than fat, so you feel full on fewer calories and eat less. For example, a study from Sweden found that women who ate a protein-carb casserole at lunch ate 12 percent less food at dinner than did women who ate only carbs for lunch. In addition, ounce for ounce, carbs and protein supply half the calories of fat, so you fill up before you fill out. Carbs provide fuel to help your body run smoothly, while protein helps maintain a constant blood sugar level, so you avoid the sugar highs and lows that tempt you to overeat. While your plate may be arrayed with vegetables, fruits, whole grains, and protein-rich lean meats or soy, you still need a little fat from oil, avocados, nuts, or seeds to make that weight-loss plan palatable, tasty, and enjoyable.

Cutting Out All Fat

Fat is fattening. A study from Vanderbilt University found that if you overeat fatty foods, you store up to 95 percent of the excess as body fat, while the equivalent in excess carbs results in a slightly lower fat conversion—85 percent of the extra calories. "Dietary fat is more readily stored as body fat, if only because the body must work harder to convert carbohydrates and protein to fat, while the dietary fat can be stored as is. That increased work equates to a slight loss of calories," says Robert H. Eckel, M.D., professor of medicine at the University of Colorado Health Sciences Center and chair of the American Heart Association's Council on Nutrition, Physical Activity, and Metabolism.

Excess is the operative word here. There is no evidence that dietary fat is stored in any greater amount than carbs or protein if you are balancing calories-in with calories-out as exercise. Overeating is what gets us into trouble, and it is much easier to overeat fat, since it is a concentrated source of calories. A wealth of research shows that high-fat diets are the ones most likely to result in piling on the pounds, mainly because they are calorie-dense. In contrast, foods rich in fiber and water—from smoothies, tomato juice, and fruit to soups, stews, veggies, and cooked whole-grain cereals—fill us up on fewer calories and are the best waist cinchers.

People on low-fat diets do reduce calories and lose weight, but they find the diets hard to stick with. A moderate-fat weight-loss diet (30 percent fat) sometimes is easier for people to follow, so dieters are more likely to keep the weight off. Several studies, including one from Purdue University, found that eating a handful of nuts a few times a week aids in weight loss.

The trick is including the right fats. Unhealthy saturated fats, such as those in bacon and cheese, along with trans fats, such as those in some margarines and snack foods, are typically found in less than nutritionally perfect foods, and they raise your risk for heart disease. You're far better off including small amounts of healthy fats from soy, nuts and seeds, olive and canola oils, avocados, and fish, which aid in weight loss, lower disease risk, and are usually found in foods that also supply hefty doses of vitamins, minerals, fiber, and phytochemicals. For example, compared with potato chips, soy nuts are packed with nutrients that lower heart-disease risk. Both salmon and red meat supply high-quality protein, but salmon also is low in saturated fat and supplies omega-3 fats that lower heart disease risk and may help prevent osteoporosis, memory loss, depression, and arthritis. Peanut butter supplies protein, B vitamins, potassium, and trace minerals, while regular old butter is just fat. By including a few healthy fats in your weight-loss plan, you'll enjoy the diet process and get more of a nutritional bang for your calorie buck.

The Low-Carb Craze

Despite the current diet buzz that carbs pack on the pounds, the truth is that carbs are not the problem. Researchers at Stanford

University School of Medicine reviewed the entire body of published research on the safety and effectiveness of low-carb diets and concluded that there is nothing magical about curtailing carbs. "Granted, low-carbohydrate diets do work, at least in the short term and especially for very overweight people, but the dieters lose weight because they cut calories, not because of a specific drop in carbohydrates," says Dena M. Bravata, M.D., M.S., lead researcher on the study. George Bray, M.D., of the Division of Obesity, Pennington Biomedical Research Center, at Louisiana State University, echoes that point: "Weight loss is not a matter of only reducing carbohydrate, any more than it is an issue of just cutting back on fat. It is the reduction in calories that results from limiting either one that matters when it comes to losing weight and maintaining the weight loss."

Moreover, the weight you lose on low-carb diets is not necessarily the right kind of weight. When you eliminate carbs, you quickly drain your body's reserves of glucose, stored as glycogen in tissues. For each gram of glycogen burned, the body loses 4 grams of water. The rapid weight loss in the first week or two of a low-carb diet is more water than fat. The first time you snack on crackers or chips, your body restocks glycogen stores, and the water weight bounces back.

Again, the drawback to carbs is that we are eating too much of the wrong stuff, gobbling record-breaking amounts of refined grains high in sugar, white flour, and fat. In contrast, replacing at least half the refined grains in your diet with fiber-rich whole grains helps keep you trim. According to researchers at Tufts University, people who load up on fiber-rich foods, such as whole grains, feel satisfied and less hungry than do people who chow down on processed grains. Adding as little as 14 grams of extra whole-grain fiber to your diet slices about 10 percent from your calorie intake, which could leave you weighing up to 4 pounds less. Here's one way to do it: have two slices of whole-wheat toast topped with peanut butter and served with orange juice for breakfast, a black bean and cheese burrito wrapped in a whole-wheat tortilla at lunch, and a side of wild rice along with your fish and vegetables at dinner. Now, how hard is that?

High-Protein Meals

Protein does aid in weight loss, but the benefits are minimal. A review of the literature by Susan Roberts, Ph.D., professor of nutrition at the USDA Human Nutrition Research Center on Aging at Tufts University, found that the metabolism-boosting effects of protein did not translate to much weight loss. She did find that high-protein diets are more satiating, so people eat less and lose weight, however: "The problem here is that there are no long-term studies on the health effects of high-protein diets, other than we know that consuming two to three times the recommended protein intake contributes to calcium loss from bone and possibly osteoporosis," says Roberts. There is no need to reinvent nutrition just to manage your weight. The best advice for long-term weight loss *and* health is to choose a low-fat, high-fiber, portion-controlled diet.

Rapid Weight Loss

If you lose more than 2 pounds a week, you're likely to lose more muscle and water than fat weight. "It takes a 3,500-calorie cut to lose a pound, so, realistically, it is impossible to lose more than 1 or 2 pounds of fat a week, because you can't cut more than 1,000 calories a day from most diets," Foreyt explains. The rest of the weight loss is water or, in cases of severe calorie restriction (as in detox diets or fasting), lean tissue such as muscle. In addition, rapid weight loss doesn't work for the long term. "All the literature shows that people who lose weight too quickly regain it just as fast," Foreyt says, adding that people typically feel so deprived on these diets that the diet pendulum eventually swings from abstinence to binge. "Besides," Kelly Brownell states, "even a perfectly planned diet can't guarantee even adequate, let alone optimal, nutrition when food intake falls below 1,200 calories a day."

You'll lose more fat and less water if you first set reasonable weight-loss goals and then create a plan to lose 1 to 2 pounds a week by making simple changes in what you eat and how much you move. "You also stack the deck in favor of maintaining the weight loss because you've learned realistic eating habits you can stick with for life," says Foreyt.

Skip Meals

Skipping meals is a big mistake, whereas eating regularly is key to weight loss. A few studies show that people who divide their food intake into little meals and snacks have an easier time managing their weight, sometimes because they take in fewer calories, other times because nibbling helps control appetite. "Eating more frequently aids weight loss, not because it speeds up metabolism, but because it helps a person deal with hunger signals," Foreyt points out. At the same time, however, other studies show that obese people eat more frequently than their leaner buddies, so obviously it's not just when, but also what, you eat that is important. "Once again, it's an issue of losing sight of the forest for the trees. Even if meal frequency has a slight advantage over the standard three square meals a day, it's insignificant if your lifestyle is not conducive to frequent snacking," says Brownell. He stresses that designing an eating plan that both maintains a desirable weight *and* fits your lifestyle is the ultimate goal.

The Salad Diet

The fact that salad dressing is the primary source of fat in women's diets attests to the confusion over what is really a healthful salad and what is a fat-laden disaster. Many fatty concoctions—croutons, pasta salad, potato salad, cheese, bacon bits, crispy noodles, and ham, just for starters—are guzzled under the guise of "salad fixings." Take, for example, the Caesar Salad with Crispy Chicken with all the fixings at McDonald's, which packs 560 calories and almost half of your day's allotment of fat (more than 32 grams, or 8 teaspoons)!

Of course, nobody gets fat by eating vegetables, and salads still are a dieter's best friend as long as the dressing is low-fat and used sparingly and the salad is built on raw and crispy produce. "Vegetables are low in calories and high in fiber, which fills you up, so it's no wonder that people who lose weight and maintain the loss base their diets on fiber-rich foods, such as vegetables," says Foreyt. Aim for two vegetables or fruits at every meal, a crispy green salad every day, and at least one vegetable at every snack.

Packaged Diet Foods

There's nothing wrong with having a packaged bar or canned shake on occasion, but if you depend on them daily, you never learn to manage your weight on real food, so the pounds reappear when you return to normal eating habits. These highly processed bars and shakes might be easy to grab, and the serving size is generally spelled out in no uncertain terms, but most are candy bars and soda pop in disguise, containing too much sugar or fat, too little fiber, and no phytochemicals.

Diet soft drinks are a different story. Theoretically, using no-calorie foods should work. Switching from cola to diet cola every day can save yourself about 160 calories, which should mean about a 17-pound weight drop in a year (160 calories × 365 days ÷ 3,500 calories in a pound). Yet, Americans guzzled $1.2 billion worth of artificial sweeteners and fat replacers in 2004 and gained weight. While there is no evidence that low-calorie foods promote weight gain, there also is no evidence that people who shift to artificial sugars and fats, without doing anything else, lose weight.

One hitch is that when people consume low-fat, sugar-reduced, low-calorie, or calorie-free foods, they compensate by eating more later. In a study from Pennsylvania State University featuring a midmorning yogurt snack, women who were told that they were snacking on reduced-fat yogurt ate more food later at their midday meal than women who were told the yogurt was full-fat, regardless of the actual fat content of the snack. To make no-calorie and low-calorie foods work for you, use them in combination with tried-and-true habits for permanent weight loss, such as controlling portions, focusing on produce, and exercising daily.

Yo-Yo Dieting

Yo-yo dieting, also called weight cycling, refers to going on and off one diet after another. First of all, according to Susan Roberts, "There's no good evidence that weight cycling does any long-term harm to metabolism or body fat distribution." Granted, metabolism slows a bit when you lose weight, but that's because you lose a little muscle that had helped support the extra fat. Drop a few pounds of muscle, and metabolism slows, by about 9 calories for every pound of muscle lost. We're also aging as we ride the diet roller coaster, so any slip in metabolism could be more a result of getting older than of dieting per se. Regardless, even if there is a slight drop in metabolism, you can make up the difference with exercise.

That said, limited evidence does suggest that yo-yo dieting might increase the risk for other health problems. In one study, yo-yo dieting elevated blood pressure, while in another study from the University of Pittsburgh, yo-yo dieting lowered HDL, the good cholesterol, increasing a woman's risk for developing heart disease. If not for your metabolism, then for your health, finding a healthy diet you can live with for life makes much more sense than reinforcing the habit of jumping onto every fad-diet bandwagon.

Kick the Habit

Kicking the fad-diet habit and losing weight for good takes a personal transformation, not just a switch to diet soda or a moratorium on chips (although that would help!). Fortunately, you've been learning how to manage your weight ever since you picked up this book. That's because the very foods that fuel your body and mind are also the foundation of a healthful weight-loss diet. Starting in the Introduction and throughout every chapter since, this book has put the kibosh on the habits that lead to weight gain, while replacing them with new habits that will help ensure a healthy body and desirable weight. For example, from previous chapters you've learned to:

- **Do it for you.** To avoid the fad-diet trap, the yo-yo diet cycle, and the inevitable gain-back phase, you must be ready to lose the weight for you, your health, your self-esteem, and your own happiness—not because your partner wants you thinner, Aunt Milly thinks you look a bit chunky, or your high school reunion is coming up. No one can do it for you, and you should do it for no one but yourself. You must stop making excuses, shuffling the blame, or putting it off, and take responsibility for your waistline and your health.

- **Get ready for a whole new you.** Changing any diet habit takes effort and always leads to new experiences, new foods, new eating patterns, and possibly even new friends, pastimes, and hobbies. You had it drummed into your head in Habit 6: Excuses, Excuses, Excuses—to be thinner, fitter, healthier, and more energetic, some things must change. Unless you are ready to ride the waves of change, you're likely to foil all your efforts to be the best that you can be and instead return to old, more comfortable patterns.

- **Accept that it won't be easy.** You must be ready for permanent change. That means the going won't always be a walk on the beach. In fact, only 25 percent of people who have successfully lost weight and maintained the loss say that the process was easy; the rest admit it was tough. The welcome news is that most of them say that maintaining is easier than losing weight, especially if the weight was lost through sensible eating and exercise.

- **Measure success.** Keep a journal, set realistic goals and minigoals, monitor your progress, and develop creative solutions to key situations. The dieters who lose weight are the ones who keep track of their behavior by logging their bites, while those who don't keep a journal are less successful and may even gain weight, according to a study in the journal *Obesity Research*.

- **Practice, practice, practice.** Any new habit—be it an eating style, an exercise schedule, or a thought process—will feel uncomfortable at first. Just keep practicing, day after day. Before you know it, that grilled chicken salad for lunch will be a treat, and you won't even miss the doughnuts in the employees' snack room.

- **Handle emotions without food.** Successful weight maintainers eat when they are truly, physically hungry and soothe anxiety, stress, loneliness, sadness, depression, and a host of other emotions with back rubs, bubble baths, walks in the woods, and other nonfood remedies.

Lose Weight Gradually

It's not that successful dieters know some secret. Every woman knows what she needs to do to drop weight: cut calories and move more. The difference is that successful dieters have figured out how to do that. They've developed the right habits and a lifelong eating plan that results in a gradual weight loss of no more than 2 pounds a week.

That's what you need to do. Strive for no fewer than 1,200 calories a day if you are short or relatively inactive (add 500 calories if you are tall and/or active). You should increase exercise, not cut calories further, if you are unable to lose weight on this low-calorie plan. A diet that falls below 1,200 calories a day (called a very-low-calorie diet, or VLCD) increases your risk for gallstones and heart problems, as well as fatigue, constipation, dry skin, and even hair loss. VLCDs are reserved for obese people and must be monitored by a physician. Even a perfect diet falls short on vitamins, minerals, fiber, healthy fats, and phytochemicals at this calorie limit, so it's essential to take a vitamin and mineral supplement to fill in some of the nutritional gaps.

How Many Calories Do I Need to Cut to Lose Weight?

You must know how many calories you currently consume before you can calculate how many you need to cut in order to lose weight. That means keeping a food journal, as discussed in Habit 1. Write down everything you eat, how much (remember to use a scale and measuring cups to accurately identify portions), and when. Tally the calories using a calorie-counting book or computerized nutrition-analysis program, to find your starting point. To make calorie counting fun, check out sites on the Web, including Calorieking, Nutritiondata, and Foodcount. Or snag a diet-diary program for your cell phone or PDA! Once you know your current calorie intake, deduct 500 calories per day to lose a pound a week.

Another means of figuring out your calorie needs requires a bit of math:

- For women between the ages of 18 and 30—multiply your weight by 6.1 and add 487, for your basic calorie needs. For women 31 to 60—multiply your weight by 4 and add 829.
- Next, multiply this basic number by 1.3, 1.5, 1.6, or 1.9, depending on whether you are sedentary, slightly active, moderately active, or very active, respectively.
- Once you have determined your current calorie intake, cut 500 calories from this total (or add 500 calories in exercise) to lose about a pound a week (a 3,500-calorie deficit = 1 pound).

John Foreyt has an even easier formula. He recommends the 100/100 plan: "To lose a couple of pounds a month, I have clients cut 100 calories from their daily diets and add 100 calories in exercise. This is as easy as eliminating the pat of butter on a slice of toast and walking 20 minutes every day."

The ABCs of Weight Loss

Dieting is not about willpower. It's not about following canned programs or set rules. The diet that will work long term for you is a product of learning what triggers you to overeat and developing new ways to manage those situations. Lena, a legal assistant in Orlando, often ate when she was home alone, especially if she was bored, tired, or parked in front of the television. The ice cream tasted great at the time, and eating it gave her something to do, but she always felt guilty and disappointed in herself afterward.

A Quick Guide to Calorie Tracking

As long as you are honest about your portions, you'll have no trouble estimating calories in real foods, such as fruits, vegetables, whole grains, nonfat and soy milk, legumes, nuts, and meats.

Category	Examples	Calories (approx.)
Vegetables	4 cups lettuce; ½ cup carrots; ¼ cup potatoes; 1 cup most other vegetables	25
Fruit	1 piece medium-size fresh; ½ cup canned; 6 ounces juice	75
Whole grains	1 slice bread; ½ bagel; ½ cup pasta, rice, or oatmeal	100
Milk products	1 cup nonfat milk or light soy milk; 6 ounces plain nonfat yogurt; 1 ounce low-fat cheese	100
Protein-rich foods	3 ounces extra-lean meat, poultry breast, or fish; ¾ cup tofu; 2 eggs; 1 ounce nuts; ⅔ cup cooked dried beans and peas	150
Fat	1 teaspoon canola oil, olive oil, butter, or margarine; 2 tablespoons low-fat dressing; 1 tablespoon mayonnaise	45

Reaching for ice cream or potato chips doesn't just happen. There is always a situation, feeling, thought, or person that entices you to eat. That "something" is called an *antecedent*. Your response to an antecedent is called the *behavior*, and the result of your behavior is called the *consequence*. These three stages in every

What's My BMI?

The body mass index (BMI), although not perfect, is a better measure of your weight than the bathroom scale, since it takes into account your height as well. Here's how to calculate your BMI, with an example of a woman who is 5'5" and weighs 135 pounds.

1. Enter your weight in pounds (135) _____
2. Multiply that number by 703 (135 × 703 = 94,905) _____
3. Multiply your height in inches by itself (65 × 65 = 4,225) _____
4. Divide the answer on line 2 by the answer on line 3 to get your BMI (94,905 ÷ 4,225 = 22.47) _____

BMI categories:
   Under 25 = normal weight
   25 to 29 = overweight
   30 and above = obese

eating episode make up the ABCs of habits. Tracking your ABCs is a simple way to get a handle on what causes you to eat too much, choose the wrong foods, or forgo exercise. As Foreyt says, "The only way to change behavior is to be aware of what you are doing."

When keeping food records, write down any antecedents (A)—the situations, time of day, thoughts, or feelings that cause you to eat inappropriately. Also, pay attention to the consequences (C) of your actions. Like Lena, do you feel guilty or angry at yourself? Does the food calm you down or relieve boredom? Does not going to the gym satisfy your urge to veg out, but later make you depressed and discouraged about your ability to stick with exercise? Pick one or two "A"s that are undermining your best intentions to eat better or exercise more. Then decide on a new behavior (a new "B"), a new habit, you will develop in its place that will have positive results. Lena decided to straddle the exercise bicycle in the evenings and pedal while watching television. The "C"s of this new habit were that she restrained from eating, fit in her daily exercise, and ended up feeling energized and happy.

Eat Low-Calorie, Low-Fat

When aiming for a new eating style that will help you take the weight off for good, keep in mind that your best bet is to cut both fat and calories. "It is a lot easier to restrict calories when you cut fat, while cutting fat aids in weight loss only if it is accompanied by a drop in calories," says Brownell. Gram for gram, fat has more than twice the calories of carbohydrates or protein. It also is more readily stored in fat tissue when consumed in excess.

That doesn't mean living a Spartan life. Low-fat fare can taste even better than fatty stuff, once you learn to spice it up with fresh ginger, cilantro, red pepper flakes, and other yummy flavors. Studies even show that once women adapt to low-fat diets, they lose their desire for fattier foods. "Once eating healthy, low-fat meals became a permanent way of life for me, the search for delicious low- or no-fat recipes got to be a hobby," says Sally, a grocery store checker in New Haven.

Successful dieters lose the weight and keep it off by limiting calories and cutting fat to about 24 percent of calories. They shy away from low-carb or fad diets and, instead, monitor calories and portions, eat lots of produce and quality carbs, and limit fat grams. "They also eat consistently, regardless of whether it's a weekday, weekend, or holiday," says Phelan. They eat at least three meals a day, and many include a few snacks, too. "Ask masters what is different about their diets today compared with the past, and they overwhelmingly respond that they used to eat haphazardly and now make a concerted effort to eat regular meals," says Fletcher. For example, 8 out of every 10 successful dieters report eating breakfast every day.

The eating plan is simple: Vegetables, fruit, breads, cereals, legumes, and pasta are mainstays of a successful dieter's eating plan, with moderate intake of nonfat milk products, chicken breast, and fish, and small amounts of extra-lean meats. Many limit or eschew visits to fast-food restaurants. The putting into practice of these guidelines varies, but everyone should tailor weight-loss efforts to accommodate the right amount of produce and quality carbs.

Focus on Produce. The starting point of any sensible weight-management eating plan is an emphasis on fruits and vegetables. Filling up on produce means that you won't have the room for calorie-dense stuff. Fruits and vegetables contain lots of water and fiber, two ingredients known to fill you up before they fill you out. These foods should constitute at least half of the foods in your eating plan. The other half will come from grains, nonfat or low-fat milk products, and extra-lean protein foods, such as chicken breast, fish, and legumes. You can spice up the menu with a few high-quality fatty foods such as nuts, nut butters, avocados, and olive oil in cooking.

Emphasize Quality Carbs. Carbohydrate-rich foods are the fuel on which your body and brain function. However, large amounts of refined carbs can cause blood sugar levels to jump, leading over time to possible problems with insulin resistance, weight gain, and even diabetes in some people. That's why you want to choose primarily quality carbs, such as whole grains (at least three a day), legumes, and starchy vegetables, including sweet potatoes. They rate lower on the glycemic index, a measure of how easily the body turns a particular food into blood sugar. Cook pasta al dente (firm, but soft), since this lowers the glycemic index score. If you do eat refined grains, limit the portion to a half-cup serving of pasta or rice, not a plate-load.

By doing this, you will automatically scale back on unnecessary calories. That's because the more processed a food, the higher its calories, fat, sugar, and/or salt and the lower its fiber, vitamins, minerals, and phytochemicals. You are aiming for the maximum nutritional return on your calorie investment, so choose the baked sweet potato, not the tater tots or french fries; the oatmeal, not the granola bar; the steamed broccoli, not the frozen broccoli in cheese sauce; and the blueberries, not the blueberry-flavored breakfast cereal. Also, consider taking a moderate-dose, well-balanced vitamin and mineral supplement.

Exercise Every Day

Any diet that says you can lose weight without sweating is lying. In a survey conducted by *Consumer Reports*, 8 out of 10 successful losers said exercise was their number one strategy for maintaining their loses. Most cited walking, while 29 percent also cited weight training. Every study on successful dieters has found the same thing. "Everyone focuses on food when it comes to weight loss, but they really should do just the opposite," says Jim Hill, Ph.D., at the University of Colorado Health Sciences Center. People should put the primary emphasis on their activity level and then eat accordingly. "Ask yourself, 'How active will I be?' and then adjust your calories to match that level of exercise," Hill advises. Not only does exercise burn calories, but it also helps regulate appetite. The more weight you have to lose, the more active you must be to reach that goal. In contrast, those people who regain their weight typically are the ones who stopped exercising and/or increased their intake of fatty foods.

You don't have to excel at kickboxing or run a marathon. Hey, you don't even have to do all your exercise at once. Start gradually. Add a 10-minute walk to your daily routine, at least five days a week. After two weeks, increase that walk to 15 minutes. Add time and increase the pace until you are walking vigorously for an hour a day, most days of the week. "I found that I have to walk every day," says Sally. "Even one day off breaks my routine, making it harder to start back up again." (For more on exercise, refer to Habit 6: Excuses, Excuses, Excuses.)

No time for an hour walk? No problem. Break it up into two 30-minute walks or even four 15-minute walks. As part of your new habit, buy a pedometer and keep track of your steps. "Aim for 8,000 to 12,000 steps a day, depending on your weight history," says Hill. Make a game of it by tracking your steps and trying to beat the numbers each day. In addition, increase your physical activity during normal living. People who don't gain back their weight spend less time sitting and watching television. They take the stairs and not the escalator, walk to the store rather than drive, get up to talk with a fellow employee rather than send an e-mail, and spend their free time moving and hardly any time vegging.

Practical, Not Perfect

Most diet successes settle for less-than-ideal bodies. "If you saw most of the masters in my study walking along the street, you

What Does a Healthy Weight-Loss Diet Look Like?

The goal is to lose no more than 2 pounds a week, while taking care of your health. That means a diet that supplies lots of vitamins, minerals, fiber, and phytochemicals, along with healthy monounsaturated fats and enough protein.

Breakfast:
⅔ cup of oatmeal cooked in 1 cup of 1 percent low-fat milk and topped with 1 tablespoon of maple syrup
Half a cantaloupe drizzled with lemon juice
Green tea

Midmorning Snack:
1 cup of low-fat, plain yogurt mixed with ⅓ cup of fresh fruit
Sparkling water with lime

Lunch:
1½ cups of lentil soup with ½ cup of frozen chopped spinach
1 slice of whole-wheat bread or 1 small whole-wheat roll
10 baby carrots
Water

Midafternoon Snack:
1 ounce of almonds
Sparkling water with lemon

Dinner:
4 ounces of grilled salmon fillet
1 medium baked sweet potato
1 cup of steamed broccoli
½ cup of cooked instant brown rice

Nutritional Analysis: 1,522 calories, 25 percent fat, 54 percent carbohydrates, 21 percent protein, 29 grams fiber, 1,253 mg calcium, 511 mcg folic acid

wouldn't say they were thin," says Fletcher. On average, the success stories in the National Weight Control Registry have lost about 29 percent of their body weight, sending them from obese to normal, not skinny. If you aim for a comfortable weight, though it may be heavier than you'd hoped, you'll be more likely to maintain it, and you'll enjoy life more than you would if you struggle to maintain an unrealistic weight on a severe diet. You'll also dramatically reduce your risk for diabetes, high blood pressure, heart disease, and joint problems.

Being practical means including a few of your favorite foods in the diet. "You are not likely to stick with an eating plan if you feel deprived," says Susan Moores, M.S., R.D., spokesperson for the American Dietetic Association. Budget in a small piece of

Weight Loss in a Nutshell

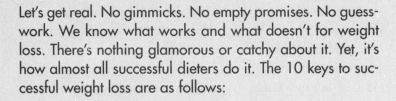

Let's get real. No gimmicks. No empty promises. No guess-work. We know what works and what doesn't for weight loss. There's nothing glamorous or catchy about it. Yet, it's how almost all successful dieters do it. The 10 keys to successful weight loss are as follows:

1. **Focus on low-fat, high-fiber foods.** Base your diet on vegetables, fruits, legumes, whole grains, and nonfat or soy milk, along with small amounts of nuts, extra-lean meats, or fish.
2. **Pare down your portions.** Huge amounts of any food will cause weight gain. Learn what reasonable portions look like (refer to Habit 3: Not Being Honest).
3. **Exercise every day.** Start small and work up to an hour of moderate exercise (the equivalent of brisk walking) daily.
4. **Set realistic goals.** Whether it is a weight goal, a diet-change goal, or an exercise goal, shoot for a practical solution, not your dream outcome.
5. **Strive for healthy, not skinny.** Eat for your body and your mind, and your weight will take care of itself!
6. **Don't let slips escalate to a relapse.** At the first sign of a 5-pound weight gain, return to record keeping, increase exercise, and/or rein in food consumption.
7. **Take charge.** Don't play the victim game by using excuses or blaming others. Accept responsibility for your weight and your health; then take action to hit your targets.
8. **Revamp your life.** You are not "on a diet"; you are creating a style of eating that you will follow for the rest of your life. That means garnering support from family and friends, finding ways to soothe your emotions

without food, and creating new pastimes that will bolster your efforts.

9. **Change your mind-set.** Believe you can do it. See yourself as fit. Feel in control. Eliminate self-defeating thoughts and replace them with messages of encouragement and empowerment.

10. **Don't deprive yourself.** Enjoy life. Have a cookie or a piece of cake. Just use common sense: treat yourself on occasion, not daily, and keep the portion small.

chocolate cake or dish of ice cream on occasion. Even have your chocolate every day—just make it two chocolate kisses, not a hefty box of candy.

Moderation is key, and defining "moderation" is even more important. "For years, I said I ate my favorite foods only once in a while, but what I really meant was that I ate one or two of my favorite foods every day. It was a handful of cookies on Monday, bacon and eggs on Tuesday, cheese pizza on Wednesday. The end result was I was overeating every day," says Sally. You need to set limits on what "moderation" and "occasional" mean. A once- or twice-a-week indulgence won't hurt your weight-loss efforts, but giving in more often than that could bring you up short.

Commit to Health

The women who are most successful at permanent weight loss are those whose chief motivator is the desire to be healthier. They've waved good-bye to the bad habit of fad dieting, and they no longer measure success just on the scale, because they realize that fitness comes first. They aren't just maintaining a weight; they are maintaining a lifestyle. They may have spent extra time counting calories or reading labels in the beginning, but they don't do that forever. In fact, successful dieters say that maintaining the weight loss takes less effort than losing the weight. Your overriding goal is to be the best and healthiest you for the rest of your life. This plan requires a firm commitment from this day forward, not to just lose weight and keep it off, but to modify habits so they support your health and, ultimately, maintain the best weight for you.

Drinking Away Our Waistlines

There's still another insidious way you could stymie all of your noble initiatives to be healthy: not by putting the wrong food on your plate, but by pouring the wrong liquid into your glass. You can faithfully watch what you eat, shying away from doughnuts at the office, rolls and butter at the restaurant, and sugar cookies at home; you can eat mindfully, only when hungry, and never off others' plates—and yet unknowingly add hundreds of empty calories to your daily menu just by sipping soft drinks and flavored sports waters during the day or alcohol at night.

A slushy margarita during happy hour, a can of cola while watching TV, or a glass of burgundy in the evening by the fireplace is such a natural accompaniment to visiting with friends or unwinding at the end of the day that we sometimes forget about the calories we are consuming. Bad move. Ignoring calories in beverages is a habit that often trumps our most earnest pursuits to be healthy or lose weight.

Silent Calories

Liquid calories accumulate fast. Our bodies don't register calories from liquids, so the calories in a cola or a gin fizz are added to, rather than replace, other calories in our total day's intake. It's as if the internal calorie-counter in the brain that tells us when we've eaten enough is oblivious to liquids' calorie load. In one study, people who drank 250 calories worth of soda, orange juice, or milk at lunch ate as much as those who drank sparkling water. In another study, from Purdue University, people were given a snack of either jelly beans or a soft drink, both having the same number of calories. Only the people drinking their calories gained weight.

It's noteworthy that liquid incorporated into food, such as a casserole or thick soup, tends to fill us up, so we eat less and are more likely to lose weight. In contrast, liquids served with a meal or downed during happy hour have no appetite-suppressing effects. This might explain why study after study shows that the more soft drinks a woman consumes, the more prone she is to gain weight. It's a direct effect: weight goes up in proportion to each can of pop.

Cola Calories

Soft drinks are a particular nemesis, since they are our leading source of sugar. We average women are guzzling 61 percent more soda today than our peers drank back in the 1970s, for a total of almost 54 gallons a year, or more than a gallon a week! At 9 to 10 teaspoons of sugar per can, that's a sizable dose of nutritionally defunct sweetened junk. A Harvard study found that people who drink soda consume about 200 more calories a day, and a study from the University of Minnesota also found that people who drink as little as 9 ounces of soda daily consume 188 calories more every day than people who don't drink these beverages. In less than three weeks, a 9-ounce-a-day person has consumed the excess calorie equivalent of a pound of body fat.

High-fructose corn sugar (HFCS) is the sole sweetener in almost all soft drinks. Our intake of HFCS has increased more than 1,000 percent since the early 1970s and now accounts for about 40 percent of the sugar we consume. This sweetener is digested, absorbed, and metabolized differently from regular sugar

The Sugar Adds Up

According to the latest statistics from United States Department of Agriculture, each woman averages up to 150 pounds of sugar a year, or about 29 teaspoons a day (some consume up to 40 teaspoons a day). Soft drinks are the foremost contributor:

Beverage	Calories	Sugar (teaspoons)
Cola—12 ounces	150	10
Sunkist orange soda—12 ounces	210	13
Mountain Dew—12 ounces	190	12

Don't think you're doing your health a favor by switching to a trendy pop or fruity drink:

Beverage	Amount	Sugar (teaspoons)
Strawberry Passion Awareness Fruitopia	20 ounces	18
Gatorade	8 ounces	3½
Arizona Original Iced Tea with lemon flavor	8 ounces	6½
Tropicana Twister Orange Raspberry	8 ounces	6½

and is more likely to make its way into fat stores. It is suspected to be a contributor to this country's growing obesity problem.

Even water can pour on the pounds. For many women, commercial waters with added vitamins, herbs, and flavorings often replace good old tap water. Hey girl, being clear doesn't mean it's calorie-free! You'd be better off getting your vitamins from a supplement and avoiding the 30 to125 calories in that overpriced bottle of workout water.

Josephine Six-Pack

"When we go out to dinner, I have a gin martini with two olives to start, and then a glass of wine with dinner. Who cares about the calories when you're drinking a delish, chilled martini!" says Nancy, an editor and writer in Los Angeles. Agreed. A drink or two on occasion is no big deal. It's the habit of making frequent trips to the bar that could tip the scales.

Alcohol is the least filling of the four calorie-containing substances. Protein is the most filling, followed by carbohydrates (such as starchy foods), fat, and, finally, alcohol. At 7 calories a gram, alcohol also has a calorie content closest to fat, so the calories shoot up. The average drink—such as a stein of beer, a glass of wine, or a shot of liquor—supplies about 150 calories, but that's just a start. When you add sugary mixes or cream to any drink, you can double or even triple the calories.

Women think of beer as fattening, but you'll gain weight twice as fast on a vodka tonic or a Cosmopolitan as on a can of beer. A 4-ounce margarita supplies about 190 calories (the calorie equivalent of eight chocolate kisses), a Brandy Alexander or Golden Cadillac adds 253 calories (the calorie equivalent of a McDonald's apple pie), a Long Island Iced Tea has 275 calories (the calorie equivalent of an order of fried onion rings), and a hot buttered rum or mint julep packs up to 300 calories a glass (the calorie equivalent of two 1-ounce bags of chips). An Apple Martini can range from 111 to 344 calories, depending on the recipe. You probably would never eat a big slice of German chocolate cake with coconut-pecan frosting before dinner, but you've just swallowed the equivalent in calories in that one drink alone. Even Nancy's regular martini is the calorie equivalent of a slice of pizza. A woman having two Apple Martinis and a glass of wine is treating herself to more calories than she would get in two Quarter Pounders! While you're at it, watch out for serving size. A pint-size margarita is four servings and close to 800 calories.

The body uses the calories in alcohol differently from the way it uses other calories. Our bodies are designed to get rid of alcohol as quickly as possible, since it's a poison that can't be stored. Alcohol is used preferentially for energy, followed by carbs, then protein, then fat. So, the fat in a Separator's half-and-half or in the steak accompanying a glass of wine, which in the absence of alcohol might be burned for energy, heads straight for storage on the thighs, hips, and waist. "A meal that includes alcohol, fatty foods, and excess calories is especially fattening, since more of those calories are stored as body fat," says Barbara Rolls, Ph.D., professor of nutrition at Pennsylvania State University and author of *The Volumetrics Eating Plan.*

The Spillover Effect

We also eat more when we drink. Alcohol stimulates appetite by increasing the production of saliva and gastric acids, both of which cause abdominal contractions that resemble a rumbling stomach. Combine that with alcohol's ability to dissolve our resolve, and you have the perfect recipe for overindulgence. In fact, we gobble as much as 200 more calories when a meal is accompanied by one alcoholic drink, compared with when we don't imbibe while eating. Even one glass of wine or beer breaks down our inhibitions, so we are more likely to take a laissez-faire approach and eat more of all the wrong stuff. "Drinks are most likely to add extra calories to the diet when they are consumed in the evening," says Rolls. There's no time to compensate by eating less later in the day, so the calories are stacked on top of your total day's intake. That's what happened to Christi, a dental hygienist in La Mesa, California, whenever she went to parties where there was a buffet. "I don't know what gets into me," she says. "I don't even like meatballs, but there I am with a glass of wine in one hand, powering down a plate of meatballs with the other."

Eating a little extra is not a deal breaker if a woman is having only a glass or two of wine a week, but Americans consumed 65.5 billion brewskis, 29.3 billion liquor drinks, and 13.7 billion glasses of wine in 1999. That averages 2.5 gallons a year for every woman, or two to five drinks a day and up to 18 percent of her calories. We're drinking outside the home more often than in the recent past, and young women are among the fastest-growing consumers of alcohol. We drink to have fun. We drink to relax. We drink to indulge ourselves, to celebrate, and to bond with friends. Nancy is probably typical: "I have a glass (sometimes two) of white wine with dinner every night. It makes the meal seem more worth sitting down to—more festive, and it's become part of our nightly dinner ritual."

We also drink more than we think. In one study, many women guesstimated that they had 3 to 11 drinks a week, only to find with record keeping that they drank two to three times that much. More than one in eight women binge (more than three drinks in one day) at least once a month. Don't get me wrong: it's fine to include a little alcohol in our lives; it might even improve health, reduce our risk for disease, and extend our lives (as discussed in the following section). Just be conscious of the fact that this habit also could detract from your nutrition and add to your waistline if you are not careful.

Cheers: Why Wine Is Good for You

A small amount of alcohol is good for your heart. It keeps the arteries clear, inhibits blood clots that can otherwise lodge in arteries, leading to heart attack and stroke, and raises the good type of cholesterol, called HDL-cholesterol. Moderate drinking also might improve bone density, lowering a woman's risk for osteoporosis, and reduce her risk for dementia in later years.

Like an apple a day, wine might be especially good at keeping the doctor away. Along with its alcohol content, wine contains a slew of health-boosting, antioxidant-rich compounds—such as phenols, flavonoids, and resveratrol—that protect arteries from inflammation and damage. Both red and white wine have health advantages, but red wine appears to have more antioxidants. These compounds prevent the bad cholesterol, LDL-cholesterol, from being damaged by oxygen fragments. Damaged LDLs are most prone to sticking to artery walls, contributing to the devel-

What Is Moderate Drinking?

Most people know what alcohol abuse looks like: Problem drinkers can't stop drinking before they become intoxicated. They may be arrested for drunk driving, drink in the morning to relieve a hangover, or be unable to recall events that happened while they were drinking. Alcohol often interferes with their lives, jobs, social and family relationships, and health. Short of those extremes, the categories can be fuzzy. Here are general guidelines:

- A light drinker has 1 drink a year to 3 drinks a week.
- A moderate drinker has 4 to 14 drinks a week.
- A heavy drinker has 15 or more drinks a week, or more than 2 drinks almost every day.

opment of atherosclerosis and heart disease. The antioxidants in wine prevent this reaction. Just as oxygen in air causes iron to rust, oxygen fragments, called free radicals, play havoc with tissues. Phenols and other compounds in wine interrupt this deadly reaction. Wine and its antioxidants also might lower the risk for dementia and macular degeneration, a major cause of vision loss, and might even extend life.

Resveratrol in red wine is especially good for you. It blocks cancer-causing substances, which encourage cells to mutate, and appears to stop already mutated cells from becoming cancerous, possibly by turning off tumor-stimulating enzymes. In addition, mutated cells already multiplying uncontrollably can be corralled and controlled by resveratrol. All told, women who drink wine in moderation also have a lower heart-disease risk.

Is it the wine or the lifestyle that gives wine drinkers the edge? Wine drinkers exercise more, eat better, smoke less, and, in general, are more likely to drink in moderation, compared with people who drink beer or liquor. Separating out which of those habits leads to a lower risk for disease is sometimes difficult. However, even purple or red grape juice protects LDLs from being damaged by free radicals, improves blood flow, and helps prevent blood clots by up to 84 percent, so there must be some truth to the research findings that wine drinkers cut their risk for heart disease by up to half.

The Dark Side of Alcohol

Alcohol is a prime example of how a little might be good for you but how more is not better. In fact, drinking too much is considerably more damaging to your health and quality of life than not drinking at all. Excessive drinking leads to inflammation of the pancreas, cirrhosis of the liver, increased risk for certain types of cancer, and a host of other health problems. Women are at particular risk for alcohol's damaging effects, for several reasons:

- Most women are smaller than men, so a similar dose has a stronger and faster effect on a woman's body.
- Alcohol is distributed throughout the watery portion of the body, but women have more body fat, which means a smaller watery compartment to hold alcohol. Consequently, alcohol concentrates faster in a smaller space than in a man's body.
- Women metabolize alcohol more slowly than do men. We have smaller amounts of alcohol dehydrogenase, the enzyme that breaks down and detoxifies alcohol before it enters the bloodstream.
- Women have a higher risk of dying in a car crash at a given blood-alcohol concentration, suggesting that alcohol has a greater impact on our driving skills than it does for men.

What it all boils down to is that alcohol rises higher and lingers longer in our systems. Women end up with a higher blood level of alcohol and are more likely to get drunk than are men from the same amount of alcohol consumed. We also are more susceptible to tissue damage from those elevated alcohol levels, causing damage to the liver, heart muscle, and brain and increased risk for breast cancer, osteoporosis, and dementia. For these reasons, women should limit their intake to one drink a day, versus two drinks a day for men.

Alcohol places a strain on our nutritional health. Even moderate drinking can flush certain nutrients out of the body and increase the body's requirement for others. For example, alcohol reduces the availability of vitamin C, increases urinary losses of potassium and calcium, and is associated with deficiencies of magnesium and zinc. Other nutrients at risk include vitamin A, vitamin B_1, vitamin B_6, vitamin B_{12}, and folic acid.

Alcohol is toxic to all tissues, and more than 60 health problems have been linked to alcohol abuse. It damages the digestive tract, heart, liver, and brain. It causes irreversible birth defects, neurological problems, and as much as a sixfold increased risk for cancers of the mouth, throat, and esophagus. Even moderate drinking might shrink two areas of the brain, possibly increasing the risk for reduced thinking ability and poor memory. One study found that while having a drink a day reduced the risk for dementia later in life, having more than two drinks a day doubled the risk. Too much alcohol also supplies empty calories, increases the risk for fatigue, aggravates depression, disrupts sleep, and can lead to addiction. Increased risk for traffic accidents, ruined families, missed work, and shattered friendships also are blatant reasons not to drink too much.

The biggest health risk for women who drink is breast cancer. The Nurses' Health Study at Harvard University, which has followed more than 89,000 women between the ages of 34 and 59, found that women who sip three to nine alcoholic drinks a week have a 30 percent higher risk for breast cancer than teetotalers. Other studies have found that after two drinks, every extra drink per day increases breast cancer risk by an additional 7 percent.

While researchers are not sure why alcohol raises cancer risk, one theory is that drinking elevates blood levels of the female hormone estrogen, which in turn jump-starts cancer cells. Cancer risk increases even more if a peri- or postmenopausal woman is on hormone replacement therapy. "Most of the known risk factors for breast cancer are beyond our control," says Susan Moores, M.S., R.D., spokesperson for the American Dietetic Association. "Any factor that can be modified, such as eliminating alcohol if you are at high risk, is especially important," she says. So, play it safe: if you have a family or personal history of breast cancer, think seriously about how much, or if, you want to drink.

You also shouldn't mix alcohol and medications, including both prescription and over-the-counter. Alcohol can enhance a drug's action, leading to greater side effects. It can cancel out or lessen a medication's effectiveness, such as in the case of antibiotics. Alcohol can convert medications to toxic chemicals that damage tissues (e.g., mixing alcohol with acetaminophen can cause liver damage). Finally, alcohol can magnify the sedative effects of certain medications, including antihistamines.

Kick the Habit

A can of soda, a glass of wine, or a beer several times a week is fine. But if you find you are drinking closer to the average for women in this country—a gallon of soft drinks a week and/or more than one alcoholic beverage daily—then you need to take a hard look at how this habit is influencing your calorie intake, your weight, and your health. Moderation is the sensible course. Soft drinks should be an occasional treat, not a daily habit. Have one or two a week, not a day. To maximize the health benefits of alcohol, such as lowering heart disease risk, and avoid the dangers of weight gain and breast cancer, women should limit alcohol to one drink a day.

The size of that drink is critical. I learned this the hard way several years ago while working with two people, Sue and Vito, for a "Good Morning America" segment called "New Year, New You" (which I mention in Habit 4). I was to help them lose weight for the New Year's kickoff and then report what worked and what didn't. In my first interview with Vito, I asked the typical questions about his daily eating habits, including how much alcohol he drank. He said he had only a drink or two a day, at most. That seemed reasonable . . . until we walked into his favorite hangout in Vail, where he was greeted by name and ushered to his regular table, and his "one drink" glass—filled to the brim with beer—was placed in front of him. The glass sat on the floor and reached chin level. It must have contained a gallon of beer! In contrast, the official "one drink" a day is 5 ounces of wine, 12 ounces of beer, or 1.5 ounces of hard liquor (80 proof). Vito's "one drink" was the equivalent of almost 11 servings!

The health benefits of wine or other alcoholic beverages also depend on when, as well as how much, you drink. A woman's risk for breast cancer increases after as few as six drinks a week. That is six drinks spread over six days, not gulped all at once. You can't drink your week's allotment of wine on Saturday and get the same health benefits as you would from controlling your daily intake. Besides, six mai tais before dinner means almost 2,000 calories, not to mention one lulu of a headache and a ton of regret the next morning.

Have your glass of wine with meals, rather than before, between, or after. "A glass of wine with a healthy meal that includes soup, salad, vegetables, lean meat, and fruit for dessert

Do You Drink Too Much?

Ask yourself the following questions. A "yes" answer to one or more could be a red flag that you are drinking too much.

— 1. Have you ever thought you needed to cut back on your drinking?
— 2. Are you annoyed by others who voice their concern about your drinking?
— 3. Do you have feelings of guilt about your drinking or your behavior when you are drinking?
— 4. Have you ever used alcohol as an eye-opener or to counter the symptoms of a hangover in the morning?

combines the ingredients needed to enhance feeling full on fewer calories," says Rolls. In contrast, drinking during happy hour makes you more likely to nosh on fatty snacks and then also eat a full meal. In short, moderate drinking with meals is less likely to increase your total day's calories, compared with drinking at other times.

Just as you should eat slowly and mindfully, you also should develop the habit of drinking slowly. It takes the liver one to two hours to detoxify the alcohol in one drink. If you drink any faster than that, alcohol accumulates in the blood and tissues. The buzz you feel means you are saturating your brain and tissues with the toxic effects of alcohol—you now have passed the point of reaping any of the health benefits of alcohol.

Nutrition and Alcohol

Even nutritionally adequate diets become inadequate with too much alcohol. But, again, you can drink in moderation without compromising your nutritional health. It's a good idea to take a moderate-dose multiple vitamin and mineral on a regular basis, and especially if you drink. Supplements can't protect the body from alcohol, but they help restore nutritional losses; the body needs the extra nutrients to repair damages caused by drinking too much. For example, vitamin E and other antioxidants curb alcohol's free-radical damage to tissues, vitamin C is needed to rebuild collagen, folic acid and other B vitamins aid in cell repair, and vitamin B_6 is required for protein building.

Folic acid is particularly important if you drink. Alcohol depletes tissues of this B vitamin, leaving cells vulnerable to cancerlike changes, which may be one of the reasons alcohol increases cancer risk. Including lots of foods rich in folic acid—spinach and other greens, orange juice, asparagus, broccoli, beans, peanuts, and fortified cereals—in the daily diet along with a supplement that contains 400 mcg of folic acid can lower some of the elevated cancer risk that comes from drinking alcohol. One study found that women who drank three glasses of wine a day had a 41 percent greater chance of developing breast cancer than nondrinkers, but that risk was offset if the women also consumed ample amounts of folic acid. Similarly, in a study on 90,000 middle-aged women, researchers found that those who had at least one drink daily and took in less than 300 mcg of folic acid had a 30 percent higher risk of breast cancer than women who drank less than one drink a day. Risk increased by only 5 percent in women who drank but also consumed more folic acid.

The 10 Rules for Drinking

1. Have no more than one or two drinks a day.
2. Never drink on an empty stomach.
3. Don't drink if there is any chance you are pregnant or if you have a history of alcoholism. Think seriously about whether you want to drink at all if you have a family or personal history of breast cancer.
4. When drinking, alternate an alcoholic beverage with a nonalcoholic beverage. For example, have a glass of wine and then drink a glass of ice water.
5. Beware of sweetened drinks: they taste great, so it's easier to overdo it.
6. Never have "one for the road." Stop drinking one to two hours before driving. Better yet, ask the designated driver to take you home.
7. When hosting a party, offer a wide selection of nonalcoholic beverages, including sparkling water, diet soft drinks, and iced tea.
8. When attending parties, take your own nonalcoholic beverage.
9. At social gatherings, choose a drink that is not your favorite. You will drink less.
10. Drink with meals, rather than before, between, or after.

Managing Key Situations

You may vow to either not drink or drink in moderation, but sometimes that is easier said than done. Most people don't like to drink alone, so the social pressure to join the crowd can be great. Toasting the birthday boy or ringing in the New Year doesn't have to mean drinking alcohol at all and certainly doesn't require getting drunk. One habit worth practicing is planning ahead of time how you will handle these key situations when the pressure or temptation to drink can overwhelm your best intentions to break this habit. That plan might include one or more of the following actions:

- Serve nonalcoholic alternatives at parties and other social events. Take your own to someone else's party.
- Pace your drinking. Plan to alternate one glass of wine with a glass of diet cola, or dilute a drink with lots of water, fruit juice, or ice.
- Think light. Do your waistline an even bigger favor by switching from regular beer to no-alcohol beer and you cut calories in half. Check labels on light beers, since they vary in calorie content.
- Nix the drinks made with high-calorie mixes, such as Lemon Drops, flavored martinis, piña coladas, and margaritas. Make your one drink a day a glass of wine and you'll save 100 or more calories in comparison.
- Dress up nonalcoholic drinks. Add zest to club soda, diet ginger ale, or other drinks by serving them in fancy glasses garnished with colorful straws and fruit wedges. Whip up elegant or gourmet nonalcoholic beverages, such as mango daiquiris using rum-flavored extract.
- Think grapes, not wine. Make nonalcoholic drinks with purple or red grape juice to get some of the health-boosting compounds found in red wine. Look for Concord grape juice that has not been diluted with white grape juice. Other foods that contain heart-healthy compounds found in red wine include

berries, plums, currants, all deep red-blue fruits, apples, onions, oranges, and grapefruit.
- Drink water, not soda pop, to quench your thirst.
- Eat well. Keep healthful snacks handy so you have something else to do with your hands and mouth besides gulp down another drink.

If you sometimes overdo it, you also need a sober-up plan. Don't count on coffee to do the trick, since all it does is liven up a groggy drunk. A walk in the brisk night air also won't magically remove alcohol from the system, since muscles don't use alcohol for energy. Bite the bullet and accept that it takes as many hours to sober up as the number of drinks consumed. The more diluted the drink and the more slowly it is sipped, the less likely it is to leave you with a hangover.

A variety of supplements with names like Hangover Helper and Drink Ease claim to cure the headache, exhaustion, and nausea of a hangover. None has been approved by the Food and Drug Administration, and all are a waste of money. The only known hangover remedies are to drink a lot of water, take a pain reliever such as aspirin, and wait it out. The best cure of all is to avoid the hangover in the first place by drinking in moderation and only on occasion.

Water: The Perfect Beverage

Water is fat-free, sugar-free, and calorie-free, and it works with, rather than against, the body's natural thirst and hunger systems. Its energy density is zero. Replace the typical 19 ounces of soft drinks guzzled daily by each American with plain water, and you will quench your thirst and siphon about 200 calories from your daily diet, the equivalent of a 1-pound weight loss every fortnight.

Water is the most important nutrient in our diets, second only to oxygen as being critical to life. Our bodies can't store excess water for future needs, so daily intakes are essential for almost all body functions, including digestion, absorption, circulation, excretion, transporting nutrients, building tissue, and maintaining body temperature.

Every system in the body—from reproduction and digestion to circulation, mood, and memory—depends on water. Water helps ward off fatigue (the number one health complaint in the United States), keeps tissues hydrated, and helps prevent headaches, kidney stones, and urinary tract infections. "Your body just won't work right without enough water. It can't rid itself of waste products, so toxins accumulate. The cells can't function properly when water balance is disrupted," according to Nancy Clark, M.S., R.D., nutrition coach at SportsMedicine Brookline, in Massachusetts. Even mild dehydration, such as losing 1 to 2 percent of body weight, results in a variety of problems, from headaches, fatigue, and weakness to light-headedness, poor stamina, reduced short-term memory, and poor concentration and reasoning ability.

Some people mistake hunger for thirst, turning to ice cream when what their bodies really want is a glass of ice water. Thirst mechanisms are different from hunger mechanisms, but many people aren't connected with their bodies' hunger signals, so they don't accurately distinguish one signal from another, mistaking hunger for thirst or fatigue. The next time you find yourself wanting to nibble but aren't really physically hungry, try drinking a glass of water and waiting 15 minutes to see if the urge to snack subsides. In one study, two out of every three people who had lost weight and maintained the weight loss said they make a concerted effort to drink water to control their weight. It tastes good, is refreshing, and helps limit food consumption. Many successful dieters also state that drinking a glass of water helps them satisfy the desire to eat between meals when they aren't really hungry.

Susan Kleiner, Ph.D., R.D., of the University of Washington, cautions that one of the first symptoms of dehydration is fatigue. People who exercise, live or work in hot climates, perspire heavily, or are pregnant or breast-feeding are at especially high risk for mild dehydration. This places stress on a woman who is trying to juggle a busy lifestyle with the additional time and emotional demands of eating healthfully or dieting. Again, it's easy to mistake fatigue for hunger and to trot off for a snack when what you really need is cool, clear water. Fatigue from being dehydrated also can wilt the determination to adhere to a diet, resulting in slips and relapse.

The average body loses about 11 cups of water daily. Many conditions escalate fluid losses beyond this mark. For example, women can sweat away a quart of water during an hour of strenuous activity, especially in hot climates, and people lose more body water at high altitudes than at low altitudes. The suggestion to aim for at least 8 glasses of water a day is a moderate and safe recommendation that can only benefit a person's health. How can you make this a habit?

- Fill a pitcher with your daily allotment of water and keep it on your desk at work or the kitchen table at home.
- Fill eight glasses with water and place them in a convenient spot, such as the kitchen counter or dining room table.
- Take eight big gulps of water every time you pass a water fountain (one slurp is approximately 1 ounce).
- Need a little incentive to drink water? Try dressing it up with a twist of lemon, lime, or orange. Or, mix a little fruit juice with sparkling water and ice.

You'll know if you are getting enough fluid when your urine is pale yellow to clear and you urinate every two to four hours. Dark yellow urine is a sign that your body is lacking in water and is trying to conserve. (One exception to this rule is if you take large doses of B vitamins, which can color the urine a bright yellow.)

Think Moderation

Alcohol, especially wine, can have some health benefits for some women. Moderate drinking also can fit easily into a plan to lose or maintain weight. When you overindulge, though, the calories mount, as can damage to tissues. So, if you choose to drink—

either alcohol or soft drinks—always exercise self-control, drink in moderation and mindfully, and remember that every calorie counts whether it comes from food or drink. That glass of red wine might slightly protect your heart, but it isn't a necessity and never is a substitute for more productive habits, such as exercise, eating right, and not smoking.

The All-or-Nothing Approach to Dieting

"Every so often, I go on food jags during which I try to eat really well. It's my feeble attempt to drop 10 pounds. I buy health foods, like wheat germ, organic broccoli, and brown rice. I exercise after work for an hour. I drink eight glasses of water every day and take my vitamins. I go all out, and I do really well for a week or so. But, then I get discouraged because I don't see results. Before I know it, I'm back to frozen dinners or takeout, and curled up on the couch eating Famous Amos chocolate chip cookies while channel surfing, instead of biking as my evening workout," says Karen, an occupational therapist in Carlsbad, California.

From a review of Karen's diet, it was clear that she didn't need to adopt a whole new lifestyle to lose the weight. All that was needed for her to lose a few pounds and feel better was to cancel her regular after-lunch frozen yogurt and stop raiding the cookie jar at night. That would lop 400 calories from her daily intake, allowing her to shave 10 pounds in three months. If she added even 10 minutes of brisk walking to her daily routine, she'd lose weight even faster and hike her energy level. Her stabs at an all-out lifestyle-overhaul were unnecessary and too extreme for any long-term success. In the final accounting, that approach actually was a liability rather than an asset, because she never did give up sweets, she continued to pack on the pounds, and she felt defeated and powerless in the face of her failure. Just like Karen, any woman with the habit of throwing herself into a diet with an all-or-nothing mentality forfeits her chances of long-term success.

Why the All-or-Nothing Mentality Fails

Most women who have struck a balance between a healthy weight and living realistically have learned to make simple changes in their lifestyles. Anne Fletcher, dietitian and author of *Thin for Life*, studied what she calls masters, people who have lost weight and successfully maintained the loss for years. "Masters put a stop to the all-or-nothing mentality of being either on or off a diet or an exercise plan. They give themselves permission to deviate from perfect, and they recognize that there are no cut-in-stone rules about eating healthy or weight control," she says. They don't punish themselves when they eat a doughnut or two or when they skip exercise for a week. They don't throw their hands up and say, "I blew it. I obviously can't do this, so I might as well give up altogether." What they do is take immediate action before the situation gets out of control.

Regardless of the vow, any all-or-nothing attempt is personal sabotage in action, including these no-no's:

- Classifying a food as either "healthy" or "junk"
- Being either "on" or "off" a diet
- Deciding to lose a specific number of pounds and nothing short of that is satisfactory
- Eliminating entire food groups, such as grains or dairy
- Labeling oneself as "good" or "bad" when it comes to eating or exercise
- Attempting a total makeover of one's diet all at once
- Committing to a two-hour intense workout every day in order to lose weight fast (having not lifted a finger in months)
- Vowing to eat no sugar (or carbs, fast food, fat, or whatever)

No one is perfect. Everyone swings and misses now and then. To leave no room for mistakes is like expecting yourself to be an Olympic athlete without training. "In an effort to lose weight, people often resort to the very eating habits that aggravate weight gain," says Wayne C. Callaway, M.D., associate clinical professor of medicine at George Washington University. All-or-nothing dieters skip meals, give up all grains, stop snacking, live on "diet" foods, or in one way or another severely restrict the types of foods they eat. "Consequently," Callaway says, "they often feel deprived, which results in the pendulum swinging from abstinence to binge." Meanwhile, reaping the benefits of healthy eating or exercise typically takes only patching the holes in a few things you're already doing. Seldom does it require a total life remodel.

All-or-Nothing and Your Weight

Have you ever decided to lose a whole bunch of weight, say 20 or more pounds, and then lost a few pounds, become discouraged, and quit? If so, join the club. Thousands of women do that every day. This all-or-nothing goal comes back to bite you in the "you know what" because it doesn't allow you to celebrate the victories along the way.

That's exactly what happened in a study from the University of Pennsylvania in which people who weighed an average of 218 pounds were asked to define their goal weights as "dream," "happy," "acceptable," or "disappointing." Most of the subjects chose a goal weight loss of 69 pounds, or about 32 percent of their body weight. They foresaw that a loss of only 37 pounds, or 17 percent of their body weight, would "not be successful at all." Yet, losing even 10 percent of body weight, which for people in this group would have been 22 pounds, can have profound effects on health—lowering the risk for high blood pressure, heart disease, diabetes, breast cancer, and more. A moderate weight loss in people with high blood pressure can eliminate the need for medication in up to half of such cases. A weight-loss equivalent of 10 percent to 20 percent of body weight in obese women can lower heart-disease risk by 40 percent or more. Even shedding a few pounds means your clothes will fit better. However, the people in this study focused only on a certain number on the scale and lost sight of the huge successes along the way.

Any woman who falls victim to the all-or-nothing mentality needs to get real. It is ridiculous for a 200-pound woman to set her goal at 130 and then feel like a failure when she reaches 145 pounds, or to reach the 130-pound target by such strict dieting that there is no way she can sustain the success for the coming years and decades. If she lost even 20 pounds by following the guidelines in this book, 95 percent of that weight would be fat weight. She would have lost the equivalent of 20 1-pound boxes of butter! Regardless, she would feel like a failure. In contrast, a woman who rewarded herself for every step taken along the way would celebrate big-time! After all, if you exercise and eat healthfully, that's a major accomplishment. If you lose 5 percent of your body weight in the meantime, that's a victory. If you start gaining weight and you stop the gain, that's admirable, too. Taking small steps is the habit that will transport you to enduring success.

Self-Talk: The Chatter Inside Your Head

Whether you buy in to the false hope of an all-or-nothing mentality or instead invest in a more realistic approach to your weight and health has a lot to do with self-talk, that ongoing conversation you have inside your head. This internal tape runs all day. It can lead to slips and relapses or can keep you directly on course, depending on whether the chatter is negative or positive.

Negative self-talk sounds something like this: "Now I've blown it," or "I can't do anything right," or "What's the use? I've failed at every attempt in the past; what makes me think I can do it this time?" This chatter usually accompanies an impossible goal, such as, "I'll not eat anything between meals ever again." Along comes the midafternoon munchies and an open bag of potato chips in the employees' lounge: your self-talk says you've had a hard day and you deserve a handful, or it says you've already blown your diet today with that chocolate kiss you stole from a workmate's desk, so you might as well eat the whole bag of chips. It's not just having the chips in sight that caused you to stumble off your diet path; the clincher is the self-talk that goes along with the chips. This slip easily becomes a total relapse as your self-talk tells you, "Hey, you ate the potato chips: the day is totally shot. You might as well eat whatever you want."

Self-talk filled with "I can't"s, "I shouldn't"s, or "I try, but . . ."s is a tip-off that you are hell-bent on making sure you never succeed. If you accept self-defeating thoughts, you always will sabotage your efforts to eat better, exercise more, or lose weight for good. "I'm-no-good" or "I-can't-do-it" thoughts also leave you feeling depressed, tired, and impotent. Your internal dialogue will either hold you back or lift you toward your goals. It either confirms that you are in control of your life or convinces you that you are a powerless victim. Which tape is playing in your head?

Here are a few more common examples of self-defeating self-talk:

- "I lost only a half pound this week. Why bother?"
- "I've gained a pound this week. Now I'll probably gain the rest back, too."
- "What's one more day of pigging out?"
- "This stupid diet spoils all my fun."
- "I tried to stick to my plan today, but everyone kept offering me food."

Positive self-talk has the opposite effect. Women who carry on a more positive conversation in their heads find the habit self-empowering. Needless to say, they also do much better at reaching their health and weight loss goals. They cope better and are more self-confident and assertive.

Kick the Habit

When you give up the all-or-nothing mentality and start reveling in small successes, you are much more prone to reach your goals and enjoy the process. First, you need to size up your weight goals to make sure they are reasonable; then you can develop a plan to prevent venial sins from morphing into eternal damnation, as well as learn some tricks for tweaking your self-talk.

Healthy Women Come in All Sizes

If you repeatedly have trouble reaching and maintaining a particular weight, perhaps that goal is unrealistic. You might be better off striving for a healthy weight, rather than a dream weight.

What is your healthy weight? It is the weight to which your body naturally gravitates and that it maintains when you eat according to the guidelines in the Introduction ("The Ultimate Diet Plan") and throughout this book, and when you exercise (at the level of a brisk walk) for at least 45 minutes a day. It's not the weight you sometimes reach and temporarily hold when starving yourself or exercising vigorously for hours a day. Of course, a healthy weight is never obese. No matter how stubbornly your body maintains a weight that is 20 percent or more above your ideal, this is not healthy, normal, or natural.

In general, a healthy weight is one at which you gain no more than 10 to 15 pounds after age 21 (assuming you were not overweight at that time), your waistline doesn't increase by more than three inches throughout the years (pregnancy excepted), and your body mass index (BMI) is between 19 and 25. (The BMI takes into account both height and weight, so it is more accurate than just a number on a scale.) A healthy weight is one that doesn't place you at increased risk for health problems, such as heart disease, high blood pressure, diabetes, and joint disorders. (Refer to Habit 8: Give Me the Quick Fix, Now! for information on how to calculate your BMI.)

A healthy weight also is one at which your excess fat is not stored around the middle. It is the deep fat, called visceral or intrabdominal fat, that lodges behind muscles and between organs that drives up your risk for heart disease, hypertension, diabetes, and possibly breast cancer. The dimply stuff on the surface, sometimes called cellulite, might not be pretty, but it is less harmful to your health. Of course, the fatter you are, the more visceral fat you will have. Neveretheless, a slightly plump woman who exercises daily can be fit with less visceral fat, while a lean couch potato can be out of shape with too much visceral fat.

Women after menopause are at particular risk for excess visceral fat. Prior to menopause, the female hormone estrogen encourages fat to be stored in the hips and thighs, where it is readily available for energy during pregnancy or breastfeeding. "When estrogen levels drop after menopause, fat is stored primarily in the subcutaneous (or under-the-skin) and visceral fat deposits," says Pamela Peeke, M.D., assistant clinical professor of medicine at the University of Maryland School of Medicine and author of *Fit Fat After Forty.* Excess calories are all the more apt to be stored as visceral fat if you smoke, drink alcohol, or are stressed. Along with giving up or managing these habits, exercise is your best bet for discouraging this type of body fat.

Handle a Slip Before It Becomes a Relapse

The all-or-nothing habit always fails, because you are likely to accept defeat the first time you drop the ball. Everybody slips up sometime. Every woman who has successfully made healthful changes in her diet, who has lost weight and kept it off, or who has changed any behavior has fallen short of the ideal a few times. The habit you want to adopt is to stop a minor slip from sending you over the edge.

Anything can cause a slip. Feelings, such as anger, grief, fatigue, fear, frustration, stress, excitement, or loneliness, can do it. Being worried or anticipating something, even something good like a job promotion, can cause you to deviate from your plan to some degree. You might resume snacking on cookies as a result of a change in routine, such as illness, travel, a holiday celebration, or premenstrual blahs. A harried life, work obligations, lack of support from family and friends, too little sleep, or too little time to relax can lead to forgoing exercise. Slip-prone moments are as varied as the women who attempt a diet or exercise change. For example:

- Lorie, a legal secretary in Chicago, walked for an hour before work every day for three months . . . until winter arrived. She didn't like walking in the dark and on snowy sidewalks, and she hadn't joined a gym, so she soon was back to snoozing the hour away rather than walking vigorously.
- Mary, an x-ray lab technician in Boston, went to her aerobics class four times a week . . . until she caught a cold and missed a week of classes; she never went back.

Both of these women could have prevented the interruption from becoming a permanent halt if they had taken action immediately.

View slips as learning experiences, not flaws in your character. They are opportunities to identify your stumbling blocks, so you can crank out a plan for the next time you're up against them. That means analyzing the slip and how you got to that point. For example, after a week of dieting, there you are suddenly, standing at the kitchen counter, fork in hand, eating apple pie out of the tin. Rather than ring down the curtain on your diet and eat the entire pie, and then sulk for days about what a weak-willed woman you are, ask yourself what preceded the pie encounter. Perhaps it was a thought, such as, "I'm dying for something sweet" or "I need a break." Maybe it was feeling frustrated or angry because your teenage son once again promised, but then conveniently forgot, to clean his room. Perhaps it was too little sleep the night before that dissolved your resolve. Think about what happened to lure you to the pie and then come up with a plan for how you can prevent a recurrence (e.g., you could burn off some of that anger or take a break with a walk instead of a binge).

Slips are not leading indicators of personal weakness or a lack of willpower, nor are they a telltale sign that you are a bad person. They are just information on what tempts you and what you need to plan for in the future. Don't overgeneralize a tiny departure from your purpose to mean that all your efforts to eat better or exercise more are worthless. Don't magnify a little slip and make it overly important, while minimizing your many successes. So, you ate a piece of cake at noon; that doesn't mean you now abandon all hope and have a platter of nachos for dinner. "Women run into trouble when they think about changes in all-or-nothing terms," says Susan Moores, M.S., R.D., spokesperson for the American Dietetic Association. "When you expect yourself to be perfect and then slip off track, it is so easy to think, 'Now I've blown my diet, so I may as well go ahead and eat.' Stop berating yourself. Instead, rededicate yourself to eating well *today*."

Self-Talk 101

Often slips are preceded by specific thoughts. Much of that self-talk is subtle. This flow of thoughts about everything that is going on throughout the day is so quiet that we often don't even know it's there. The first step in creating an internal dialogue that eschews the all-or-nothing mentality and supports your efforts to feel great, look fantastic, be healthy, and/or lose weight is to start monitoring what you say to yourself about these endeavors. Listen up to what tapes run through your mind about the following subjects:

- Your appearance
- Your weight
- Your ability to lose weight and maintain the loss
- Your image of yourself as an exerciser
- Your potential to be fit
- Your general health both today and in the future
- Your chances of eating well and feeling great for the rest of your life
- Food, calories, and eating in general

Take one week to open your ears to your thinking. Write down any common thoughts or themes that you detect. What do you tell yourself about life and your efforts throughout the day?

- When you stand in front of the mirror, what thoughts run through your head about your body shape, weight, looks, or aging process? For one woman, all that the mirror—and her mind—reflected was the problem areas. "Thoughts about my body in the mirror are mostly along the lines of: Wow, look what having two kids in two years does to a body! My belly has a perpetual three-months-pregnant shape, my hips are definitely wider, and the breasts are heading south."

- When standing behind a young, beautiful blonde in the checkout line, or when flipping through a fitness or fashion magazine, what thoughts about yourself are in the back of your mind? "I am constantly comparing myself with other women. When the women are bigger than I am, I feel better. When they are fit, more muscular, sexier, or slimmer than I am, I think back to my last resolution to lose weight and think that I could have looked that good if I'd stuck with it. That just makes me mad at myself," says Shannon, a health care worker in Reno.

- At parties, buffets, restaurants, and other social eating situations, what thoughts about food are influencing your choices? Victoria, a writer and mother of two in Beaverton, Oregon, has to watch the excuses that flow along her stream of consciousness. "At parties," she says, "I'll tell myself, 'I'll just have this one appetizer or sweet.' Once the floodgates open, though, I eat and eat. There's no stopping it. What started out as one taste ends up being more like a dozen."

Keep in mind that all self-talk is self-prophecy in action. Our thoughts literally program us for failure or success. Self-defeating or self-demeaning thoughts will create failure. Thoughts that you are helpless to change, that you don't have the willpower to make a difference in your life, or that you never can stick with anything long enough to see results are thoughts filled with sadness; they are self-fulfilling prophecies that lead you to make decisions and choices by which you once again fail and feel depressed. Negative self-talk always, always, always works against you. Obviously, this is not the type of self-talk you want to generate! Encouraging thoughts—especially when they are repeated throughout the day, over and over, day after day—lift us up, motivate us to stick with it, and help us reach any goal we set. They also enhance our mood and raise our energy level.

What Are You Thinking?

After a week of monitoring your thoughts, consider which patterns are helping and which ones are hurting your progress. Does your self-talk generally encourage and support health, or do negative thoughts keep you from exercising or choosing the blueberries instead of the chocolate ice cream? Does self-talk about being self-conscious of your not-quite-perfect body keep you from joining the gym, so you stay home and watch reality TV instead? Do thoughts that you'll never lose weight or be healthy precipitate your evening binges?

How does your self-talk measure up to your weight-loss goals? Are you telling yourself that you can lose the weight, you are in control of your choices, and every day gets easier? Or, are your thoughts generally centered on how miserable you are when you're eating like this, how much you hate to exercise, and how the whole process is just too hard? You will succeed at losing weight for good only if your thoughts are in line with your goals and behaviors. If they aren't, it's time to make some changes in what thoughts you allow into your noggin.

As you listen to your internal dialogue, ask yourself whether your thoughts are even accurate. As outlined in previous chapters, we are not always honest with ourselves and others about what we eat and how much we exercise. We also can be masters at fashioning excuses for why we are powerless to change. More often than not, these thoughts are not valid, yet they are potent influencers of our actions. "I only had a bite of that hamburger at lunch, so I can have extra mashed potatoes tonight" sounds reasonable, but is it valid? Not if that bite was half the sandwich and the extra helping of mashed potatoes will send you over your day's calorie limit. "I hate it when my husband brings pizza home. I have no willpower to resist it once it is in the house": is that line of thinking based in truth? Is there absolutely nothing you can do except overeat pizza and blow your diet? If you think long and hard, I bet you'll come up with a dozen alternatives that might work to resist this temptation, including having one piece of pizza and a huge tossed salad; asking your husband to bring home a small or medium-size pizza that he can finish, with no leftovers; or going for a longer walk that day so you can have the extra calories in one or two slices.

Thought Stopping

Once you have identified thought patterns that are undermining your weight and health goals, you need to stop those negative thoughts or replace them with encouraging, positive, and empowering ones. One technique is to use thought stopping. Every time you catch a negative thought in your mind, visualize a stop sign or silently tell yourself to "stop." To get your attention, mentally scream, "*Stop!*" Then consciously replace the negative thought with a productive one. For example, Halie, a college student, was tempted by her friend's french fries and found herself rationalizing that she deserved a fistful of fries because she'd had a rough day. She caught the thought just as her hand was reaching for a fry and said to herself, "Stop it!" She then replaced the destructive thought with, "I deserve to feed myself with real, quality food that will nourish me and help me reach my goals. I choose to snack on the baby carrots I brought from home, not those greasy fries loaded with calories and trans fats."

Some positive self-talk can become a mantra you repeat to yourself throughout the day. "I am becoming healthier every day" or "Weight loss is within my control" can be a message you deliver to yourself while standing in line, driving to work, sitting at your desk, or just before you go to sleep at night. Write your favorite self-talk mantras on a piece of paper and post them on the mirror, refrigerator, computer screen, dashboard, or anywhere else you are likely to see the reminder several times a day. Make sure your positive self-talk has special meaning for you and contradicts an old self-destructive tape you've played in your head in the past.

Replace Those Negative Thoughts

Say good-bye to the habit of negative self-talk and hello to encouraging and motivating thoughts:

Negative self-talk: I lost only a half pound this week. I'm never going to lose the weight.
Positive self-talk: My weight loss may be slow this week, but it's steady, and I'm going to lose the weight for good this time.

Negative self-talk: I don't have time to exercise for a whole hour, so I might as well not exercise at all.
Positive self-talk: Any amount of exercise is better than nothing. I'll do 15 minutes now and 15 minutes later this afternoon.

Negative self-talk: I can't believe I ate that piece of cake. What a loser! I can't do anything right.
Positive self-talk: I have been doing really well on my new eating plan. So what if I had that cake. I learned that skipping breakfast makes me more likely to eat sweets later in the day, so I'll start over tomorrow and make sure I save five minutes to have my cereal before leaving the house in the morning.

Negative self-talk: I tried so hard and only lost a half pound. This whole diet thing isn't worth it. I'll never lose the weight.
Positive self-talk: I am eating healthier and feeling better. That's a reward in itself. I know that weight lost slowly is more likely to stay off, so I'll just keep following my plan. I know I'll be healthier in the long run.

continued

Negative self-talk: I can't prepare healthy meals at home because my kids will complain.
Positive self-talk: I will prepare healthy foods at home and will also offer the kids their favorite foods on occasion. Everyone will be healthier as a result.

Negative self-talk: I have to cut my calories so low that I'm starving in order to lose weight.
Positive self-talk: I will continue monitoring my portions and load my plate with vegetables until I get a handle on how many calories I'm really eating. I know I can lose weight and still feel satisfied.

Negative self-talk: I can't eat after sunset or all the calories will turn to fat.
Positive self-talk: It's the total calories throughout the day that matters, not when they are eaten. I can have a healthy snack in the evening as long as I've budgeted it into my eating plan.

Negative self-talk: I would exercise if I only had more time.
Positive self-talk: Exercise is a priority. I make time for it every day.

Negative self-talk: When people tell me I look good, I think, "They are just being nice. I look awful."
Positive self-talk: I do look good and am getting healthier every day.

Negative self-talk: That girl is so much prettier than I am and so thin. I need to lose more weight.
Positive self-talk: I am exercising every day and eating healthy food. I am doing so much better at my diet and exercise than I did this time last year. I am the best I can be and feel good about that.

Negative self-talk: I'm 2 pounds heavier this week than I was last week. I'm such a slob.
Positive self-talk: Weight fluctuates day to day because of fluid changes. That weight might not be fat weight, but I will start keeping a journal again to make sure I'm not slipping up.

Negative self-talk: I can't have sweets. They go right to my hips.
Positive self-talk: I can have small amounts of my favorite foods on occasion. I plan them into my daily menu and enjoy every bite!

Negative self-talk: I should never eat fast food or carbs.
Positive self-talk: An occasional fast-food meal won't hurt me, and carbs are an important fuel for my body, especially if I choose moderate amounts of healthy ones.

Negative self-talk: If I didn't have roommates, I wouldn't have all this junk food around.
Positive self-talk: I am in control of my food choices and decide what I will eat and what I don't want to eat.

Exercise: It's Not an All-or-Nothing Proposition

Are you out of breath after walking up a flight of stairs? Is carrying the groceries from the car more tiring than it used to be? Does crossing the street to make a green light feel like running the 100-yard dash? Are you stiff in the morning? Tired in the evening? Does an afternoon of gardening leave your muscles sore for days? If so, the likely reason is that you are out of shape—you're not keeping your muscles and joints young by exercising them regularly.

Sitting on your duff won't do you in when you're 10, 15, or even 20 years old, but your muscles will take a nosedive somewhere around the 30-year mark. People lose approximately 1 percent to 2 percent of muscle mass every year after this point, which equates to a 5- to 10-pound loss of muscle for every decade. The loss usually doesn't become noticeable until the forties roll around, when you discover that pushing a door open takes two hands instead of one, or you unconsciously take the elevator to avoid even a two-story climb up the stairs. If you don't start weeding your fitness garden now, you will watch the pounds slowly proliferate, aging before your time, and risking a bunch of diseases down the stretch, including heart disease, diabetes, high blood pressure, and more. This is not a habit you want to continue, and establishing take-it-or-leave-it goals for fitness could keep you from doing what needs to be done.

Every study to date shows that both disease risk and muscle strength are dramatically improved when exercise is included in the daily routine, regardless of the woman's age or health condition. Staying fit equates to drastically lowering your disease risk and living longer. Women who continue to exercise in their second 50 years are as fit as, or even fitter than, sedentary women who are 20 to 30 years younger. This may explain why they also live longer. In fact, the more calories a woman expends in exercise each week, the longer she is likely to live disease-free and at a desirable weight.

You've read it numerous times in previous chapters: you must exercise regularly if you want to lose weight and, more important, maintain the weight loss. John Foreyt, Ph.D., director of the Nutrition Research Center at Baylor College of Medicine and an expert on weight management, found in his studies that women who exercise are the least likely to relapse. He divided people into three groups: diet-only, diet-and-exercise, and exercise-only. The exercise-only group maintained the best weight loss and reported a heightened sense of well-being. In contrast, Foreyt says the feeling of deprivation and the rigid restrictions of the dieting groups probably contributed to their failure. The bottom line? "It's better to put your efforts into healthy eating and regular exercise, than to go on rigid, all-or-nothing fad diets," says Foreyt.

I repeat: exercise is not an all-or-nothing affair. You don't have to win the Tour de France or even join a gym. You do need to move at least 45 minutes most days of the week. Divide that routine as follows:

- Aerobic activity (such as walking, swimming, or jogging, at least four hours a week)
- Strength training (such as lifting weights or calisthenics like sit-ups, at least twice a week)
- Warming up and cooling down (such as stretching, for 5 minutes before and after exercise)

Make it fun. If you are a social creature, walk with a group, play tennis, or join an aerobics class. If you need time alone to de-stress, you can jog, ride a bike, or walk the dog.

Give Yourself Some Slack

You might strive for healthier eating or a slimmer waistline, but the real goal that underlies any diet and exercise effort is to ultimately feel great and enjoy life more. Finding a balance between your dream goals and living life is an ongoing process, not an obsession. One study found that 86 percent of women admitted they postponed something, including shopping, dating, and sex, until they had lost more weight and reached their goals. Sad to say, most women don't ever get there, and they miss out on a lot of living in the meantime. You don't want to put off getting on with life in the hope that you'll first lose a few extra pounds. Time passes so fast, and life is far too short. To obsess over your weight or your health to the point of not fully embracing life could mean you will all of a sudden be 85 years old and still worrying about losing that last 5 pounds. How absurd is that!

Improving your weight and your health is not an end in itself; it is a means to an end. The ultimate goal is embracing a passionate, vital life with more energy, greater self-esteem, fewer inhibitions and fears, and a stronger feeling of freedom to be you. It includes getting more out of life, taking chances, stretching limits. Being healthy and at a healthy weight could even mean going back to school, getting the job you always wanted, traveling, hiking, volunteering your time, in-line skating, rock climbing, joining a local theater group, singing in the choir, or learning to swing dance. Striving to be the healthiest you is not about fixing your gaze on an all-or-nothing goal, but rather having the energy and drive to enjoy new interests, hobbies, pleasures, and activities. That ultimate goal is squeezing the most out of life, not waiting until you've lost 5 pounds so you can start living!

Accept yourself. Hey, even celebrate yourself! Give yourself permission to be not quite perfect. Love your flaws as you gently strive to change them. Allow a few treats in life. Talk to yourself lovingly. Pick yourself up when you fall short of your goals, and keep your eye on your triumphs, not your shortcomings.

Simple Steps, Big Results

- Don't sabotage your best efforts to be healthy and lose weight.
- Take responsibility for your life and your health.
- Focus on simple steps to reach your goals.

Those three main messages in this book are the solution to every habit that interferes with your goals to feel and look your best. We often are our own worst enemies, declaring that we want to lose weight, eat better, or have more energy, and all the while continuing to nibble off others' plates, manufacture excuses for why we don't have time to exercise, blame others for our eating habits, or jump onto the latest fad-diet bandwagon, all of which divert us from our goals.

The 10 habits discussed in this book are subtle, often invisible. Like well-worn slippers, they're comfortable, almost second nature, so we don't even notice them. As a result, we try and fail to reach one diet milestone after another, blame our lack of willpower, or contend that we've tried everything and nothing works, while those subtle habits are the true cause of our unsuccessful attempts.

Healthy and fit living doesn't take a total life overhaul. It doesn't even take major changes in what you eat or how much you move. It does require a change in priorities. All of us are living reflections of our priorities. A woman will never quit emotional eating if stuffing her feelings with food is a priority. A woman who puts others' needs before her own will have a tough time not eating mindlessly. Riding the fad-diet roller coaster of losing weight and regaining it will be a woman's life as long as the quick fix is her goal. She probably will struggle to lose weight despite eating healthy, if big portions or her daily colas or martinis are too precious to give up. On the other hand, when health is a priority, women exercise and eat well, swear off tobacco, and learn to manage their stress. A woman will spend time with family members and help them take care of themselves if they are her priority. She will go to the dentist if dental health and a pretty smile are priorities. She will adopt lifelong healthy eating habits if losing weight and maintaining the loss means enough to her.

I admit that I'm a bit prejudiced here. I believe health is the number one priority, since it is an essential brick in the foundation of a vital, passionate life. As Barbara Cartland, the British author, once said, "I consider myself an expert on love, sex, and health. Without health, you can have very little of the other two." It is difficult to get the most out of life, relish the freedom that being fit gives you, and have the energy to do all that you want when you are not in tip-top health. Of course, health is more than just the absence of disease; it's the freedom to live life to its fullest.

The fact that you are reading this book suggests that you want good health or a trimmer figure to be a priority. But is it a priority? No matter what you say is important to you, it's where you direct your attention, spend your time, and put your effort that speaks the loudest about what is most essential to you in life.

Take a moment to reflect on your priorities. Use "My Mission Statement," as provided in this chapter, to clarify how you want health and your figure to fit into your life. Only if they head your priority list will you take the time and effort to change one or more of the 10 habits that impede your efforts.

You may find from filling out your mission statement that health is not a priority right now. Perhaps you have more pressing issues at the top of your list. Maybe you are a single, working mom with young kids at home, which can make it tricky, but not impossible, to exercise as much as you would like or eat as well as you want. Maybe you are in the midst of a job change or are moving to a new city and need to settle into this new life

My Mission Statement

Describe below what a perfect day five years from now would look like. What would you be doing? How would you spend your time, and with whom? How do you look, feel, and think? How is your health? How active are you? Be specific and realistic. This is a fantasy, but also an opportunity to visualize how you could make that fantasy a reality.

_____

_____

_____

From the scene you described above, identify five major priorities in your life, such as family, health, work, where you live, climate, home, or hobbies.

1. _____

2. _____

3. _____

4. _____

5. _____

Are you spending time today on these priorities? If so, how do you incorporate them into your daily life today? If not, create a plan to include them in your daily and weekly "to do" list. What do you need to change in your life today to bring it more into line with those things that are most important to you?

before you can tackle a diet adjustment. If you are already maxed out, with no time to take on another task, don't add to your stress or set yourself up for defeat. Put major health goals on the back burner for now, and reevaluate your priorities when life settles down. However, if your blood pressure or cholesterol has gone up, if you are well above a desirable body weight, or if other serious and treatable health issues are keeping you from living well, then health must be a top priority *now*.

Even if your mind tells you that health is a priority, your heart might not be in it. Before you go for any change, evaluate how committed you are to taking the plunge. Complete the accompanying quiz—"Is Now the Right Time for a Change?"—to check your level of commitment to developing new habits at this time.

The Salami Principle: Simple Steps

Living healthy doesn't need to suck up extra time. It is more a matter of using your time more efficiently and effectively. As mentioned in Habit 6: Excuses, Excuses, Excuses, most of us waste a lot of time every day. Organizing our day and using our time more efficiently helps launch our priorities into action. People good at time management find it easier to take care of themselves and keep the weight off. A study from Kaiser Permanente, in Oakland, California, found that women who successfully lost weight and maintained the weight loss were much more likely to confront problems directly and were more self-reliant and organized than were relapsers. Women who make health a priority organize their days so they have time to exercise, prepare a healthy home-cooked meal in the evening, or fix a veggie platter to take to a party. They schedule exercise dates on their calendars as if they were doctor's appointments that cannot be missed. They keep the kitchen stocked so it is easy to prepare healthful meals in minutes. They also follow the Salami Principle for getting things done.

The Salami Principle goes like this: Even the most ardent salami lover probably couldn't eat an entire 12-inch-long salami in one sitting. However, almost anyone can finish it off by dividing that salami into a hundred thin slivers and having one or two slices every day. As the old saying goes: "You can eat an elephant if you do it one bite at a time."

Getting organized means approaching your long-term health goals as if they were that salami or that elephant. Break them into little, simple steps that add up over time to major changes in what you eat, how much you move, and how lean and fit you are. Once you go from understanding what being healthy involves to actually living it step by step, there will be no going back. You'll feel too good to settle for less.

Hundreds of simple steps have been offered throughout this book. You are the best expert on which ones will work for you. There is no cookie-cutter approach to eating well and losing weight, so don't be surprised if the simple steps you choose are different from those selected by someone else. You might come to see that if you overeat when you're tired, just having a bowl of whole-grain cereal instead of a cup of coffee in the morning is a simple step that could help cure emotional eating. Likewise, taking five minutes to have a small bowl of soup before a party could be the simple step that helps you resist the temptation to overeat at social gatherings. Put a stop to mindless eating (you won't solve world hunger by eating your kids' leftovers anyway!) and you might find that those last 5 pounds just drop off. Take the stairs instead of the escalator, include one more vegetable in your daily diet, store trigger foods in hard-to-reach cupboards, hold a glass of water in your dominant hand at parties so you are less likely to nibble, split an entree at restaurants, or switch from frying in oil to using a nonstick pan with cooking spray. Ministeps such as these nudge you toward being a healthier you. That last step alone—frying smart—will save you about 100 calories each time. Repeat that one simple step over the course of one month, and you will lose 1 pound. The "Healthy-Habits Pyramid" shown here summarizes and organizes the habits that will help ensure that you are victorious in reaching any health goal you set.

Make simple steps even easier by combining them with other items on your "to do" list. When you ride a bike with a friend,

Is Now the Right Time for a Change?

Health or weight loss might rank high on your priority list, but is this really the best time for a habit change? On a scale of 1 to 5 (1 = not at all, 5 = more so than ever), answer the following questions:

___ 1. Compared with dieting attempts in the past, how committed are you to sticking with it this time?

___ 2. How determined are you to make a habit change now and sticking with it until you reach your health goals?

___ 3. Long-term habit change requires effort. How willing are you to take the time and make the effort to reach your goals?

___ 4. Changing any habit is a step-by-step, gradual effort. For example, you should lose no more than 2 pounds a week if your goal is permanent fat loss. Are your goals to change a habit in a given amount of time realistic?

___ 5. Can you count on getting support for your habit-change efforts from friends, family, coworkers, and other important people in your life?

___ 6. Learning new habits is like learning any new skill—it requires time. Do you have time to make permanent changes in your life?

Scoring:

< 17 points: Reflects a low commitment to habit change and a high likelihood of failure. Wait, and try another time.

17 to 23: Reflects a moderate commitment to habit change, but you still need to work on motivation.

24+: Reflects high motivation. This could be the best time to change a bad habit.

you link exercising with socializing, just as you can by walking with a coworker to brainstorm work-related projects, rather than sitting in the conference room to accomplish the same task. Mend clothes, put photographs in an album, or ride your exercise bike while watching television; you'll get those pesky chores done, watch your favorite show, and keep yourself from snacking. If you regularly relax on Sunday mornings with a cup of coffee, use that time to leisurely plan your meals for the week. (Then make your week's shopping list, go to the grocery store once, and save yourself hours of time and stress from repeated last-minute trips later in the week.)

Stay positive about the habit-change process. Often simple steps toward your ultimate health goals are not about what you *can't* have, but what you *can* have. On a day-to-day basis, that means having more fruits and vegetables, such as topping your frozen yogurt with fresh strawberries, adding extra broccoli to your pasta dishes, or having a big tossed salad before you eat a meal. If you wolf down your food, it might mean making room in your meal plan for more "slow foods," which are foods that

Healthy-Habits Pyramid

You can eat healthy and lose unwanted pounds just by replacing the habits that undermine your efforts with the new habits presented in this book. The "Healthy-Habits Pyramid" reflects that. The three tiers are equally important but are ordered in terms of what to do first, with the bottom tier representing steps you should take at the outset, followed by day-to-day tips in the middle tier and then the fine-tuning tips at the top. All the tips within each tier likewise are equally important, so choose which ones work best for you. Select the tips from each tier that pertain to you. Focus on these in designing your personalized get-healthy program.

continued

**Fine-
tune
the plan:**

Eat regularly.

Eat out
with caution.

Nip weight gain
in the bud.

Cut back on excess
calories from sugar and fat.

Think before you drink
(beverages have calories, too!).

**The day-to-day plan:
Practice, practice, practice:**

Eat mindfully.

Stay motivated.

Encourage support.

Exercise for at least 45 minutes.

Eat only when physically hungry.

Convert negative self-talk to positive self-talk.

Adopt a low-fat, fiber-rich diet based on vegetables, fruits, whole
grains, legumes, and nonfat milk products.

Closely monitor your progress with food records,
portion awareness, and specific plans.

Make your own food choices; don't let others make them for you.

Preplanning steps for success:

Believe you can succeed.

Accept that there are no quick fixes.

Acknowledge that it won't be easy.

Take responsibility: Be honest. No more excuses.

Set realistic goals. (Develop a plan you can live with for life.)

take longer to eat, such as hot tomato soup; spicy foods that can't be gulped; or artichokes that must be eaten one leaf at a time. It might mean placing a big bowl of baby carrots or grapes on your desk at work so you nibble more of these and keep your fingers out of your coworkers' tempting bag of chips.

The Ultimate Goal

On a grander scale, taking care of yourself means you'll have more energy, more joy, more health, and a longer life. You'll have an easier time managing your weight, lower disease risks, better memory as you age, and a more even, upbeat mood. Hey, you might even look younger!

Simple Steps

Make many of the simple steps offered throughout this book, as well as others that complement your goals, regular habits. For example:

- Make exercise fun. Listen to books on tape, walk the dog, read a book on the exercise bike, or vary your workouts with the season.
- Eat two fruits and/or vegetables at every meal and one at every snack. You'll meet your daily quota of five to nine servings, feel full, and automatically cut back on fat and calories.
- Take a little hike every hour: If you don't have time for an hour workout, set your watch alarm on the hour and take a 5-minute brisk walk around the office. Over the course of an eight-hour shift, you'll accrue 40 minutes of exercise.

continued

- Eat regularly. If you skip a meal to save calories or as penance for overindulging the night before, you'll be more than likely to overeat later in the day.
- Brush your teeth after a meal. This helps signal the body that you're done eating and curbs the cravings for dessert.
- Turn off the tube. Hours of television watching are directly proportional to weight gain. Go for an after-dinner walk, ride the exercise bike, do laundry, or paint the living room instead.
- Just say no. Listen to your body and eat only when you're hungry, not because the food is there or because someone offers it.
- Eat slowly. This allows the food to digest and gives the stomach time to tell the brain it's full.
- Drink first. We often confuse thirst with hunger, diving for the ice cream when it's water our bodies need. Drink a glass of water and wait 15 minutes before giving in to a craving. You may find that the hunger subsides.
- Challenge yourself. If you're comfortable walking at a moderate pace, go up a short hill during your next walk, or pick up the pace.
- Be a lark. Exercise in the morning so you don't spend the rest of the day making up excuses for why you can't exercise.
- Be an expert. Learn to read labels, and purchase mostly foods that contain no more than 3 grams of fat for every 100 calories (or approximately 30 percent fat calories).
- Doggie-bag it. Most restaurant servings are platters, not portions. Put half the serving in a doggie bag for tomorrow's lunch.
- Eighty-six the fat-free desserts. Ounce for ounce, most fat-free desserts are just as calorie-dense as the higher-fat versions. Even if they are low-calorie, you aren't

giving yourself a leg up by eating the whole box. Stick to the serving size on the label.

- Eat less. Cut your typical portions of everything except vegetables and fruits by a fourth.
- Hang out with exercisers.
- Remember that the calories in beverages count, especially gourmet coffee drinks, fruit juices, and smoothies.
- Remember that every tablespoon counts. A tablespoon of mayo on a turkey sandwich, for example, doesn't seem like a lot, but over the course of one year, that daily mayo equals 10½ pounds of excess body fat.
- Don't assume you can exercise away anything you eat. A café mocha is the calorie equivalent of a one-hour jog.
- Get enough sleep. You're more likely to overeat and choose all the wrong foods (candy, chocolate, sugar, caffeine) when you're tired.
- Purchase a step counter. This small device that straps to your ankle is a great incentive to boost the number of steps you take every day.
- Eat breakfast. People who eat breakfast are much less likely to overeat later in the day. A healthful breakfast takes only five minutes and is as simple as juice, fruit, and cereal.
- Take foods with you. Pack one snack for every four hours you'll be gone. Pack your briefcase, glove compartment, or desk drawer at work with oranges, apples, yogurt, bread sticks, string cheese, and other quick-fix healthful snacks.
- Divide your plate. Fill three-fourths of your plate with vegetables, grains, beans, and fruits; the remainder can be extra-lean meat or nonfat milk or milk products. Said another way, take three bites of plant-based foods for every mouthful of meat or milk.

continued

- Drink water. Meet your daily quota of six to eight glasses, curb appetite, and possibly avoid late-night cravings by keeping bottled water in the refrigerator or filling a container with eight glasses of water and drinking one glass every one to two hours.
- Cut 100 calories each day. Lose one pound a month by simply replacing that candy bar with an orange and a banana, the ½ cup of granola with 2 cups of Cheerios, or the ½ cup of frozen broccoli in cheese sauce with ½ cup of steamed fresh broccoli.
- Take a supplement. Your vitamin and mineral needs remain the same no matter what your calorie intake. A broad-range multiple vitamin and mineral supplement will fill in the nutritional gaps on those days when calories drop below 2,000.
- Focus on health, not your waistline. When you eat for health, you are automatically adopting the best weight-management diet in the world. Successful diets fit easily into your daily routine, nourish your body and soul, and please your taste buds.
- Use time-savers. Buy precut and bagged lettuce for a salad, baby carrots for a stew, precut fruit for a snack, and prepared hummus as a dip or sandwich spread; steam frozen plain vegetables for dinner.
- Cut out or limit alcohol. Alcohol stimulates appetite and erodes your willpower. Limit wine, beer, or other alcoholic beverages to special occasions. Serve these beverages in small glasses, and intersperse alcohol with calorie-free beverages.
- Get rid of it. If those brownies or homemade cookies beckon to you, get rid of them . . . now! Give them to a neighbor, take them to the office, or throw 'em out.
- Add beans. Healthy salads and soups are more satisfying and will help curb hunger pangs longer if you add a handful of kidney beans, 3 ounces of grilled chicken breast, or other stick-to-the-ribs items.

- Sweeten with spice. Use sweet-tasting spices—such as cinnamon, nutmeg, and vanilla—rather than sugar in desserts and snacks to add flavor but no calories.
- If you can't live with it, don't buy it. Just say no to tempting foods at the grocery store if they are likely to impel you to indulge at home. Also, store tempting foods out of sight.
- Close the menu. Ask the waiter for low-calorie items, such as steamed vegetable platters, grilled-chicken salads, or sliced tomatoes. Or, order from the soup, salad, and low-fat appetizer sections and skip the entrees altogether.
- Go spicy. Overeating and food cravings can be an underlying search for flavor. Add chilies to chicken sandwiches, salsa to scrambled eggs, or curry to sauces. Try hot cuisines, such as Thai, Szechuan, or Indian.
- Stay busy. Keep your hands busy by sewing, manicuring your nails, addressing envelopes, or exercising during your crave-prone times of day, such as when you're watching TV or even when you're reading.
- Eat when you're comfortably hungry and stop when you're comfortably full.
- At parties, eat only the foods you really like.
- Clean out the kitchen. Throw away the junk, such as chips, toaster pastries, and soft drinks.
- Shop for groceries from a list to minimize impulse purchases.
- Savor one sinfully delicious dessert a week, rather than one every day.
- Switch from white bread to 100 percent whole-wheat bread and from white rice to brown rice.
- Use spinach or romaine in salads instead of iceberg lettuce.
- Double up. Double the serving size of all vegetables.

continued

- Switch from full-fat to 1 percent milk, saving 40 calories for every serving.
- Limit fast-food meals, such as burgers, fries, and fried chicken, to once a week at the most.
- Order salad dressing on the side at restaurants. Dip the fork lightly into dressing before taking a bite of salad. Plan on using only 10 percent of the dressing served.

What can great health or weight loss bring to your life? What are your ultimate goals once you eliminate one or more of those 10 habits and, as a result, get fit or lose the extra pounds? Take a few minutes and fill out the "My Life Goals" form on page 267. This list can help motivate you to be faithful to your health plan.

During the course of my 25 years in the field of nutrition, I have had the opportunity to work with hundreds of people, helping them, one step at a time, make improvements in their eating habits. I'm always amazed at how grateful the body is for a little kindness. Feed it right and move it more, and it responds tenfold. Eat well—it pays off! After following a few of the suggestions in this book, every woman—even healthy women who exercise reasonably regularly and try to eat well—says: "I never knew I could feel this good!"

As Hugh Mullegan, the Associated Press correspondent, aptly said, "What I do today is important because I am exchanging a day of my life for it." My wish for you is that you develop healthy habits that allow you to spend each moment of your precious time on Earth in great health, free and eager to embrace life to the fullest.

My Life Goals

Make a list of at least a dozen things you've always wanted to do. Rate each one on a scale from 1 to 5, with 1 being "definitely possible" and 5 being "definitely impossible." For example, my list includes learning to fly an airplane and living in New York City. I rate the pilot goal as a 2, since there is nothing stopping me except saving the money. The NYC goal is a 5 right now until my kids are grown, but the score could improve after that, as long as I stay healthy and capable of the move. Create your list and rate each item, and then choose one or two items that received a 1 or 2 score and decide how you will accomplish this goal in the near future.

I've always wanted to:	Score (1–5)	My plan to make this happen:
_____	_____	_____
_____	_____	_____
_____	_____	_____
_____	_____	_____
_____	_____	_____
_____	_____	_____
_____	_____	_____

Selected Reading

Brownell, K. *Food Fight: The Inside Story of the Food Industry, America's Obesity Crisis, and What We Can Do About It.* New York: McGraw-Hill, 2003.

————. *The LEARN Program for Weight Management 2000.* Dallas: American Health Publishing, 2000.

Fletcher, A. *Thin for Life: 10 Keys to Success from People Who Have Lost Weight and Kept It Off.* Boston: Houghton Mifflin, 2003.

Hill, J. *The Step Diet: Count Steps, Not Calories, to Lose Weight and Keep It Off Forever.* New York: Workman Publishing, 2004.

Mellin, L. *The Solution: Six Winning Ways to Permanent Weight Loss.* New York: Regan Books, 1997.

Nash, J. *Maximize Your Body Potential: 16 Weeks to a Lifetime of Effective Weight Management.* Palo Alto: Bull Publishing, 1986.

Nelson, M. *Strong Women Eat Well.* New York: G. P. Putnam's Sons, 2001.

Rolls, B. *The Volumetrics Eating Plan.* New York: Harper Collins, 2005.

Rolls, B., and R. Barnett. *Volumetrics: Feel Full on Fewer Calories.* New York: Harper Collins, 2000.

Satter, E. *How to Get Your Kid to Eat . . . But Not Too Much.* Palo Alto: Bull Publishing, 1987.

Somer, E. *Nutrition for Women.* 2nd ed. New York: Owl Books, 2002.

————. *The Origin Diet.* New York: Owl Books, 2001.

————. *Food & Mood.* 2nd ed. New York: Owl Books, 1995.

Somer, E., and J. Williams. *The Food & Mood Cookbook.* New York: Owl Books, 2004.

Stuart, R., and B. Jacobson. *Weight, Sex, and Marriage.* New York: W. W. Norton & Co., 1987.

References

Introduction

Arjmandi. B., D. Khalil, B. Smith, et al. Soy protein has a greater effect on bone in postmenopausal women not on hormone replacement therapy, as evidenced by reducing bone resorption and urinary calcium excretion. *J Clin End* 2003;88:1048–1054.

Ball, K., W. Brown, and D. Crawford. Who does not gain weight? Prevalence and predictors of weight maintenance in young women. *Int J Obes* 2002;26:1570–1578.

Bazzano, L., J. He, L. Ogden, et al. Legume consumption and risk of coronary heart disease in U.S. men and women. *Arch In Med* 2001;161:2573–2578.

Bowman, S., S. Gortmaker, C. Ebbeling, et al. Effects of fast-food consumption on energy intake and diet quality among children in a National Household Survey. *Pediatrics* 2004;113:112–118.

Bowman, S., and B. Vinyard. Fast-food consumption of U.S. adults: Impact on energy and nutrient intakes and overweight status. *J Am Col N* 2004;23:163–168.

Byrne, S. Psychological aspects of weight maintenance and relapse in obesity. *J Psychosom Res* 2002;53:1029–1036.

DeMoreno, A., and G. Perdigon. Yogurt feeding inhibits promotion and progression of experimental colorectal cancer. *Med Sci Monit* 2004;10:BR96–BR104.

Dohm, F., J. Beattie, C. Aibel, et al. Factors differentiating women and men who successfully maintain weight loss from women and men who do not. *J Clin Psychol* 2001;57:105–117.

Frazao, E., ed. *America's Eating Habits: Changes & Consequences.* ERS. USDA, Agriculture Information Bulletin Number 750. Washington, D.C., 1999.

Gorin, A., S. Phelan, R. Wing, et al. Promoting long-term weight-loss control: Does dieting consistency matter? *Int J Obes* 2004;28:278–282.

Jacobs, D., M. Pereira, K. Meyer, et al. Fiber from whole grains, but not refined grains, is inversely associated with all-cause mortality in older women. *J Am Col N* 2000;19:S326–S330.

Jiang, R., J. Manson, M. Stampfer, et al. Nut and peanut butter consumption and risk of type 2 diabetes in women. *J Am Med A* 2002;288:2554–2560.

Kasum, C., K. Nicodemus, L. Harnack, et al. Whole-grain intake and incident endometrial cancer. The Iowa Women's Health Study. *Nutr Cancer* 2001;39:180–186.

Kennedy, E., J. Ohls, S. Carlson, et al. The Healthy Eating Index: Design and applications. *J Am Diet A* 1995;95:1103–1108.

Kral, T., L. Roe, and B. Rolls. Combined effects of energy density and portion size on energy intake in women. *Am J Clin N* 2004;79:962–968.

Krebs-Smith, S., L. Cleveland, R. Ballard-Barbash, et al. Characterizing food intake patterns of American adults. *Am J Clin N* 1997;65(suppl):1264S–1268S.

Krebs-Smith, S., and L. Kantor. Choose a variety of fruits and vegetables daily: Understanding the complexities. *J Nutr* 2001;131:487S–501S.

Kritz-Silverstein, D., D. Von Muhlen, E. Barrett-Connor, et al. Isoflavones and cognitive function in older women: The Soy and Postmenopausal Health in Aging (SOPHIA) study. *Menopause* 2003;10:189–190.

Lara, J., J. Scott, and M. Lean. Intentional misreporting of food consumption and its relationship with body mass index and psychological scores in women. *J Hum Nutr Diet* 2004;17:209–218.

Liu, S., J. Manson, M. Stampfer, et al. A prospective study of whole-grain intake and risk of type 2 diabetes in U.S. women. *Am J Pub He* 2000;90:1409–1415.

Putnam, J., J. Allshouse, and L. Kantor. U.S. per capita food supply trends. More calories, refined carbohydrates, and fats. *FoodReview* 2002;25:2–15.

Scagliusi, F., V. Polacow, G. Artioli, et al. Selective underreporting of energy intake in women: Magnitude, determinants, and effect of training. *J Am Diet A* 2003; 103:1306–1313.

Wien, M., J. Sabate, D. Ikle, et al. Almonds versus complex carbohydrates in a weight-reduction program. *Int J Obes* 2003;27:1365–1372.

Wyatt, H., O. Grunwald, C. Mosca, et al. Long-term weight loss and breakfast in subjects in the National Weight Control Registry. *Obes Res* 2002;10:78–82.

Habit 1

Bellisle, F., R. McDevitt, and A. Prentice. Meal frequency and energy balance. *Br J Nutr* 1997;77:S57–S70.

Bro, R., L. Shank, T. McLaughlin, et al. Effects of a breakfast program on on-task behaviors of vocational high school students. *J Educ Res* 1996;90:111–115.

Compa Nicklas, T., L. Myers, and G. Berenson. Total nutrient intake and ready-to-eat cereal consumption of children and young adults in the Bogalusa Heart Study. *Nutr Rev* 1995;53:S39–S45.

Drummond, S., N. Crombie, and T. Kirk. A critique of the effects of snacking on body-weight status. *Eur J Clin N* 1996;50:779–783.

Edelstein, S., E. Barrett-Connor, D. Wingard, et al. Increased meal frequency associated with decreased cholesterol concentrations; Rancho Bernardo, CA, 1984–1987. *Am J Clin N* 1992;55:664–669.

Fabry, P. Metabolic consequences of the pattern of food intake. In *Handbook of Physiology: The Alimentary Canal.* Sec. 6, vol. 1, 31–49.

Farshchi, H., M. Taylor, and I. Macdonald. Regular meal frequency creates more appropriate insulin sensitivity and lipid profiles compared with irregular meal frequency in healthy lean women. *Eur J Clin N* 2004;58:1071–1077.

Fogteloo, A., H. Pijl, F. Roelfsema, et al. Impact of meal timing and frequency on the 24-hour leptin rhythm. *Horm Res* 2004;62:71–78.

Gold, P. Role of glucose in regulating the brain and cognition. *Am J Clin N* 1995;61(suppl):987S–995S.

Hall, J., et al. Glucose enhancement of performance on memory tests in young and aged humans. *Neuropsychologia* 1989;27:1129–1138.

Hammond, G., and G. Chapman. The nutritional role of breakfast in the diets of college students. *J Can Diet* 1994; 55:69–74.

Hayashi, K., T. Hayashi, S. Iwanga, et al. Laughter lowered the increase in postprandial blood glucose. *Diabetes Care* 2003;26:1651–1652.

Hill, G. The impact of breakfast, especially ready-to-eat cereals, on nutrient intake and health of children. *Nutr Res* 1995; 15:595–613.

Jenkins, D., A. Khan, A. Jenkins, et al. Effect of nibbling versus gorging on cardiovascular risk factors: Serum uric acid and blood lipids. *Metabolism* 1995;44:549–555.

Jenkins, D., A. Ocana, A. Jenkins, et al. Metabolic advantages of spreading the nutrient load: Effects of increased meal frequency in non-insulin-dependent diabetes. *Am J Clin N* 1992;55:461–467.

Jenkins, D., T. Wolever, V. Vuksan, et al. Nibbling versus gorging: Metabolic advantages of increased meal frequency. *N Eng J Med* 1989;321:929–934.

Kanarek, R. Psychological effects of snacks and altered meal frequency. *Br J Nutr* 1997;77(supplement):S105–S118.

Keim, N., M. Van Loan, W. Horn, et al. Weight loss is greater with consumption of large morning meals and fat-free mass is preserved with large evening meals in women on a controlled weight-reduction regimen. *J Nutr* 1997;127:75–82.

LeBlanc, J., and I. Mercier. Components of postprandial thermogenesis in relation to meal frequency in humans. *Can J Physl* 1993;71:879–883.

Lloyd, H., P. Rogers, D. Hedderley, et al. Acute effects on mood and cognitive performance of breakfast differing in fat and carbohydrate content. *Appetite* 1996;27:151–164.

Manning, C., et al. Glucose effects on memory and other neuropsychological tests in elderly humans. *Psychol Sci* 1990;1:307–311.

McGrath, S., and M. Gibney. The effects of altered frequency of eating on plasma lipids in free-living healthy males on normal self-selected diets. *Eur J Clin N* 1994;48:408–415.

Metzner, H., D. Lamphiear, N. Wheeler, et al. Relationship between frequency of eating and adiposity in adult men and women in the Tecumseh Community Health Study. *Am J Clin N* 1977;30:712–715.

Powell, J., P. Franks, and N. Poulter. Does nibbling or grazing protect the peripheral arteries from atherosclerosis? *J Cardio Risk* 1999;6:19–22.

Schlundt, D., J. Hill, T. Sbrocco, et al. The role of breakfast in the treatment of obesity: A randomized clinical trial. *Am J Clin N* 1992;55:645–651.

Smith, A., A. Centrex, A. Maben, et al. Effects of breakfast and caffeine on cognitive performance, mood, and cardiovascular functioning. *Appetite* 1994;22:39–55.

Stubbs, R., M. van Wyk, A. Johnstone, et al. Breakfasts high in protein, fat, or carbohydrates: Effect on within-day appetite and energy balance. *Eur J Clin N* 1996;50:409–417.

Habit 2

Ball, K., W. Brown, and D. Crawford. Who does not gain weight? Prevalence and predictors of weight maintenance in young women. *Int J Obes* 2002;26:1570–1578.

Binkley, J., J. Eales, and M. Jekanowski. The relation between dietary change and rising U.S. obesity. *Int J Obes* 2000; 24:1032–1039.

Bovbjerg, V., B. McCann, D. Brief, et al. Spouse support and long-term adherence to lipid-lowering diets. *Am J Epidem* 1995;141:451–460.

Bove, C., J. Sobal, and B. Rauschenbach. Food choices among newly married couples: Convergence, conflict, individualism, and projects. *Appetite* 2003;40:25–41.

DeCastro, J., E. Brewer, D. Elmore, et al. Social facilitation of the spontaneous meal size of humans occurs regardless of time, place, alcohol, or snacks. *Appetite* 1990;15:89–101.

Devine, C., and C. Olson. Women's perceptions about the way social roles promote or constrain personal nutrition care. *Women Heal* 1992;19:79–95.

Guthrie, J., B. Lin, and E. Frazao. Role of food prepared away from home in the American diet, 1977–78 versus 1994–96: Changes and consequences. *J Nutr Ed B* 2002;34:140–150.

Herman, C., N. Fitzgerald, and J. Polivy. The influence of social norms on hunger ratings and eating. *Appetite* 2003; 41:15–20.

Jeffery, R., and S. French. Epidemic obesity in the United States: Are fast foods and television viewing contributing? *Am J Pub He* 1998;88:277–280.

Jeffery, R., and A. Rick. Cross-sectional and longitudinal associations between body mass index and marriage-related factors. *Obes Res* 2002;10:809–815.

Kahn, H., D. Williamson, and J. Stevens. Race and weight change in U.S. women: The roles of socioeconomic and marital status. *Am J Pub He* 1991;81:319–323.

Kant, A., and B. Graubard. Eating out in America, 1987–2000: Trends and nutritional correlates. *Prev Med* 2004;38: 243–249.

McKie, L., R. Wood, and S. Gregory. Women defining health: Food, diet, and body image. *Health Ed Res* 1993;8:35–41.

Meltzer, A., and J. Everhart. Self-reported substantial one-year weight change among men and women in the United States. *Obes Res* 1995;3:123S–134S.

Millen, B., P. Quatromoni, D. Gagnon, et al. Dietary patterns of men and women suggest targets for health promotion: The Framingham Nutrition Studies. *Am J H Pro* 1996;11:42–52.

Neumark-Sztainer, D., P. Hannan, M. Story, et al. Family meal patterns: Associations with sociodemographic characteristics and improved dietary intake among adolescents. *J Am Diet A* 2003;103:317–322.

Oygard, L., and K. Klepp. Influences of social group on eating patterns: A study among young adults. *J Behav Med* 1996;19:1–15.

Parham, E. Enhancing social support in weight-loss-management groups. *J Am Diet A* 1993;93:1152–1156.

Price, C. Sales of meals and snacks away from home continue to increase. *FoodReview* 1998;Sept–Dec:28–30.

Rauschenbach, B., J. Sobal, and E. Frongillo. The influence of change in marital status on weight change over one year. *Obes Res* 1995;3:319–327.

Sobal, J., B. Rauschenbach, and E. Frongillo. Marital status changes and body weight changes: A U.S. longitudinal analysis. *Soc Sci Med* 2003;56:1543–1555.

Stroebele, N., and J. DeCastro. Effect of ambience on food intake and food choice. *Nutrition* 2004;20:821–838.

Habit 3

Becker, W., and D. Welten. Underreporting in dietary surveys: Implications for developmental food-based dietary guidelines. *Pub He Nutr* 2001;4:683–687.

Black, A., and T. Cole. Biased over- or underreporting is characteristic of individuals whether over time or by different assessment methods. *J Am Diet A* 2001;101:70–80.

Blundell, J. What foods do people habitually eat? A dilemma for nutrition, an enigma for psychology. *Am J Clin N* 2000;71:3–5.

Brug, J., P. van Assema, G. Kok, et al. Self-rated dietary fat intake: Association with objective assessment of fat, psychosocial factors, and intention to change. *J Nutr Educ* 1994;26:218–223.

Fisher, J., B. Rolls, and L. Birch. Children's bite size and intake of an entree are greater with larger portions than with age-appropriate or self-selected portions. *Am J Clin N* 2003; 77:1164–1170.

Foreyt, J., and G. Goodrick. Attributes of successful approaches to weight loss and control. *Appl Prev P* 1994;3:209–215.

Frobisher, C., and S. Maxwell. The estimation of food portion sizes: A comparison between using descriptions of portion sizes and a photographic food atlas by children and adults. *J Hum Nutr Diet* 2003;16:181–188.

Gilsenan, M., and M. Gibney. Assessment of the influence of energy underreporting on intake estimates of four food additives. *Food Addit Contam* 2004;21:195–203.

Goris, A., E. Meijer, and K. Westerterp. Repeated measurement of habitual food intake increases underreporting and induces selective underreporting. *Br J Nutr* 2001;85: 629–634.

Goris, A., and K. Westerterp. Improved reporting of habitual food intake after confrontation with earlier results on food reporting. *Br J Nutr* 2000;83:363–369.

Harnack, L., R. Jeffery, and K. Boutelle. Temporal trends in energy intake in the United States: An ecologic perspective. *Am J Clin N* 2000;71:1478–1484.

Heitmann, B., L. Lissner, and M. Osler. Do we eat less fat, or just report so? *Int J Obes* 2000;24:435–442.

Hill, R., and P. Davies. The validity of self-reported energy intake as determined using the doubly labeled water technique. *Br J Nutr* 2001;85:415–430.

Johansson, L., K. Solvoll, G. Bjorneboe, et al. Under- and overreporting of energy intake related to weight status and lifestyle in a nationwide sample. *Am J Clin N* 1998; 68:266–274.

Jonnalagadda, S., D. Bernardot, and M. Dill. Assessment of underreporting of energy intake in elite female gymnasts. *Int J Sport N* 2000;10:315–325.

Lara, J., J. Scott, and M. Lean. Intentional misreporting of food consumption and its relationship with body mass index and psychological scores in women. *J Hum Nutr Diet* 2004;17:209–218.

Matthiessen, J., S. Fagt, A. Biltoft-Jensen, A. Beck, et al. Size makes a difference. *Pub He Nutr* 2003;6:65–72.

McGuire, M., R. Wing, M. Klem, et al. What predicts weight regain in a group of successful weight losers? *J Cons Clin* 1999;67:177–185.

Mela, D. Consumer estimates of the percentage of energy from fat in common foods. *Eur J Clin N* 1993;47:735–740.

Mendez, M., S. Wynter, R. Wilks, et al. Under- and overreporting of energy is related to obesity, lifestyle factors, and food group intake in Jamaican adults. *Pub He Nutr* 2004;7:9–19.

Mertz, W. Food intake measurements: Is there a "gold standard"? *J Am Diet A* 1992; 92:1463–1465.

Nielsen, S., and B. Popkin. Patterns and trends in food portion sizes, 1977–1998. *J Am Med A* 2003;289:450–453.

Novotny, J., W. Rumpler, J. Judd, et al. Diet interviews of subject pairs: How different persons recall eating the same foods. *J Am Diet A* 2001;10:1189–1193.

Paisley, C., H. Lloyd, P. Sparks, et al. Consumer perceptions of dietary changes for reducing fat intake. *Nutr Res* 1995;15: 1755–1766.

Pikholz, C., B. Swinburn, and P. Metcalf. Underreporting of energy intake in the 1997 National Nutrition Survey. *NZ Med J* 2004;117:U1079.

Poppitt, S., D. Swann, A. Black, et al. Assessment of selective underreporting of food intake by both obese and nonobese women in a metabolic facility. *Int J Obes* 1998;22:303–311.

Rolls, B. The supersizing of America: Portion size and the obesity epidemic. *Nutr Today* 2003; March–April.

Rolls, B., E. Morris, and L. Roe. Portion size of food affects energy intake in normal-weight and overweight men and women. *Am J Clin N* 2002;76:1207–1213.

Rozin, P., K. Kabnick, E. Pete, et al. The ecology of eating: Smaller portion sizes in France than in the United States help explain the French paradox. *Psychol Sci* 2003; 14:450–454.

Samuel-Hodge, C., L. Fernandez, C. Henriquez-Roldan, et al. A comparison of self-reported energy intake with total energy expenditure estimated by accelerometer and basal metabolic rate in African American women with type 2 diabetes. *Diabet Care* 2004;27:663–669.

Shilts, M., M. Horowitz, and M. Townsend. Goal setting as a strategy for dietary and physical activity behavior change: A review of the literature. *Am J He Pro* 2004;19:81–93.

Tonstad, S., C. Gorbitz, M. Sivertsen, et al. Underreporting of dietary intake by smoking and nonsmoking subjects counseled for hypercholesterolaemia. *J Intern Med* 1999; 245:337–344.

Voss, S., A. Kroke, K. Klipstein-Grobursch, et al. Obesity as a major determinant of underreporting in a self-administered food frequency questionnaire: Results from the EP Potsdam Study. *Z Ernahrungswiss* 1997;36: 229–236.

Wadden, T., R. Vogt, G. Foster, et al. Exercise and the maintenance of weight loss: One-year follow-up of a controlled clinical trial. *J Cons Clin* 1998;66:429–433.

Weber, J., P. Reid, K. Greaves, et al. Validity of self-reported energy intake in lean and obese young women, using two nutrient databases, compared with total energy expenditure assessed by doubly labeled water. *Eur J Clin N* 2001;55:940–950.

Williamson, D. Dietary intake and physical activity as "predictors" of weight gain in observational, prospective studies of adults. *Nutr Rev* 1996;54:S101–S109.

Young, L., and M. Nestle. Variation in perceptions of a "medium" food portion: Implications for dietary guidance. *J Am Diet A* 1998;98:458–459.

————. The contribution of expanding portion sizes to the U.S. obesity epidemic. *Am J Pub He* 2002;92:246–249.

————. Expanding portion sizes in the U.S. marketplace: Implications for nutrition counseling. *J Am Diet A* 2003; 103:231–234.

Habit 4

Albertson, A., and R. Tobelmann. Consumption of grain and whole-grain foods by an American population during the years 1990 to 1992. *J Am Diet A* 1995;95:703–704.

Ascherio, A., M. Katan, P. Zock, et al. Trans-fatty acids and coronary heart disease. *N Eng J Med* 1999;340:1994–1998.

Bazzano, L., M. Serdula, and S. Liu. Dietary intake of fruits and vegetables and risk of cardiovascular disease. *Curr Atheroscler Rep* 2003;5:492–499.

Bendich, A. Biological functions of dietary carotenoids. *Ann NY Acad* 1993;691:61–67.

Block, G., and B. Abrams. Vitamin and mineral status of women of childbearing potential. *Ann NY Acad* 1993; 678:244–254.

Bray, G., S. Nielsen, and B. Popkin. Consumption of high-fructose corn syrup in beverages may play a role in the epidemic of obesity. *Am J Clin N* 2004;79:537–543.

Brug, J., S. Debie, P. van Assema, et al. Psychosocial determinants of fruit and vegetable consumption among adults: Results of focus group interviews. *Food Qual P* 1996;6:99–107.

Cao, G., S. Booth, J. Sadowski, et al. Increases in human plasma antioxidant capacity after consumption of controlled diets high in fruit and vegetables. *Am J Clin N* 1998;68:1081–1087.

Casto, B., L. Kresty, C. Kralyl, et al. Chemoprevention of oral cancer by black raspberries. *Anticancer Res* 2002; 22:4005–4015.

Charlton, K., P. Wolmarans, and C. Lombard. Evidence of nutrient dilution with high sugar intakes in older South Africans. *J Hum Nutr Diet* 1998;11:331–343.

Chu, Y., J. Sun, X. Wu, et al. Antioxidant and antiproliferative activities of common vegetables. *J Agric Fd Chem* 2002;50:6910–6916.

Collins, B., A. Horshka, P. Hotten, et al. Kiwifruit protects against oxidative DNA damage in human cell and in vitro. *Nutr Cancer* 2001;39:148–153.

Dittus, K., V. Hillers, and K. Beerman. Benefits and barriers to fruit and vegetable intake: Relationship between attitudes and consumption. *J Nutr Educ* 1995;27:120–126.

Eichholzer, M., J. Luthy, F. Gutzwiller, et al. The role of folate, antioxidant vitamins, and other constituents in fruit and vegetables in the prevention of cardiovascular disease: The epidemiological evidence. *Int J Vit N* 2001;71:5–17.

Forastiere, F., R. Pistelli, P. Sestini, et al. Consumption of fresh fruit rich in vitamin C and wheezing symptoms in children. SIDRIA Collaborative Group, Italy. *Thorax* 2000;55:283–288.

Gibney, M., M. Sigman-Grant, J. Standton, et al. Consumption of sugars. *Am J Clin N* 1995;62:178S–194S.

Guthrie, J., and J. Morton. Sources of added sugars in the diets of Americans. *FASEB J* 1999;13:A695.

Hagdrup, N., E. Siomoes, and R. Brownson. Fruit and vegetable consumption in Missouri: Knowledge, barriers, and benefits. *Am J Heal B* 1998;22:90–100.

Harder, B. Proof of burden. *Sci News* 2003;163:120.

He, K., F. Hu, G. Colditz, et al. Changes in intake of fruits and vegetables in relation to risk of obesity and weight gain among middle-aged women. *Int J Obes* 2004;28:1569–1574.

Herraiz, T., and J. Galisteo. Tetrahydro-beta-carboline alkaloids occur in fruits and fruit juices. Activity as antioxidants and radical scavengers. *J Agric Food* 2003;51:7156–7161.

Hou, D. Potential mechanisms of cancer chemoprevention by anthocyanins. *Curr Mol Med* 2003;3:149–159.

Hung, H., K. Joshipura, R. Jiang, et al. Fruit and vegetable intake and risk of major chronic disease. *J Natl Canc* 2004; 96:1577–1584.

Ikken, Y., P. Morales, A. Martinez, et al. Antimutagenic effect of fruit and vegetable ethanolic extracts against N-nitrosamines evaluated by the Ames test. *J Agric Food Chem* 1999;47:3257–3264.

Jenkins, D., C. Kendall, A. Marchie, et al. The garden of Eden: Plant-based diets, the genetic drive to conserve cholesterol, and its implications for heart disease in the 21st century. *Compt Bio Physl* 2003;136:141–151.

Jenkins, D., C. Kendall, D. Popovich, et al. Effect of a very-high-fiber vegetable, fruit, and nut diet on serum lipids and colonic function. *Metabolism* 2001;50:494–503.

Joseph, J., N. Denisova, G. Arendash, et al. Blueberry supplementation enhances signaling and prevents behavioral deficits in an Alzheimer disease model. *Nutr Neurosci* 2003;6:153–162.

Joshipura, K., F. Hu, J. Manson, et al. The effect of fruit and vegetable intake on risk for coronary heart disease. *Ann Int Med* 2001;134:1106–1114.

Key, T., M. Thorogood, P. Appleby, et al. Dietary habits and mortality in 11,000 vegetarians and health-conscious people: Results of a 17-year follow-up. *Br Med J* 1996; 313:775–779.

Krebs-Smith, S., L. Cleveland, R. Ballard-Barbash, et al. Characterizing food intake patterns of American adults. *Am J Clin N* 1997;65:1264–1268.

Krebs-Smith, S., A. Cook, A. Subar, et al. U.S. adults' fruit and vegetable intakes, 1989 to 1991: A revised baseline for the Healthy People 2000 Objective. *Am J Pub He* 1995;85: 1623–1629.

Krebs-Smith, S., F. Cronin, D. Haytowitz, et al. Food sources of energy, macronutrients, cholesterol, and fiber in diets of women. *J Am Diet A* 1992;92:168–174.

Krebs-Smith, S., J. Heimendinger, B. Patterson, et al. Psychosocial factors associated with fruit and vegetable consumption. *Am J He Pro* 1995:10:98–104.

Krebs-Smith, S., and L. Kantor. Choose a variety of fruits and vegetables daily: Understanding the complexities. *J Nutr* 2001;131:487S–501S.

Landrigan, P., B. Sonawane, D. Mattison, et al. Chemical contaminants in breast milk and their impacts on children's health: An overview. *Env He Persp* 2002;110: A313–A315.

Lechner, L., J. Brug, and H. de Vries. Misconceptions of fruit and vegetable consumption: Differences between objective and subjective estimation of intake. *J Nutr Educ* 1997;29: 313–320.

Lyons, M., C. Yu, R. Toma, et al. Resveratrol in raw and baked blueberries and bilberries. *J Agric Food* 2003;51:5867– 5870.

Martin, K., M. Failla, and C. Smith. Beta-carotene and lutein protect HepG2 liver cells against oxidant-induced damage. *J Nutr* 1996;126:2098–2106.

Masrizal, M., D. Giraud, and J. Driskell. Retention of vitamin C, iron, and beta-carotene in vegetables prepared using different cooking methods. *J Food Qual* 1997;20:403– 418.

Moeller, S., P. Jacques, and J. Blumberg. The potential role of dietary xanthophylls in cataract and age-related macular degeneration. *J Am Col N* 2000;19:522S–527S.

Motohashi, N., Y. Shirataki, M. Kawase, et al. Cancer prevention and therapy with kiwifruit in Chinese folklore medicine: A study of kiwifruit extracts. *J Ethnopharmacol* 2002;81:357–364.

Newby, P., D. Muller, J. Hallfrisch, et al. Dietary patterns and changes in body mass index and waist circumference in adults. *Am J Clin N* 2003;77:1417–1425.

Papas, M., E. Giovannucci, and E. Platz. Fiber from fruit and colorectal neoplasia. *Canc Epidem B* 2004;13:1267–1270.

Patterson, B., G. Block, W. Rosenberger, et al. Fruit and vegetables in the American diet: Data from the NHANES II survey. *Am J Pub He* 1990;80:1443–1449.

Persky, V., R. Chatterton, L. van Horn, et al. Hormone levels in vegetarian and nonvegetarian teenage girls: Potential implications for breast cancer risk. *Cancer Res* 1992; 52:578–583.

Poulsen, M., and J. Andersen. Results from the monitoring of pesticide residues in fruit and vegetables on the Danish market, 2000–2001. *Food Addit Contam* 2003;20: 742–757.

Pronczuk, A., Y. Kipervarg, and K. Hayes. Vegetarians have higher plasma alpha-tocopherol relative to cholesterol than do nonvegetarians. *J Am Col N* 1992;11:50–55.

Putnam, J., J. Allshouse, and L. Kantor. U.S. per capita food supply trends: More calories, refined carbohydrates, and fats. *FoodReview* 2002;Winter:2–11.

Rampersaud, G., L. Bailey, and G. Kauwell. National survey beverage consumption data for children and adolescents indicate the need to encourage a shift toward more nutritive beverages. *J Am Diet A* 2003;103:97–100.

Rissanen, T., S. Voutilainen, and J. Virtanen. Low intake of fruits, berries, and vegetables is associated with excess mortality in men. *J Nutr* 2003;133:199–204.

Rock, C., J. Lovalvo, C. Emenhiser, et al. Bioavailability of beta-carotene is lower in raw than in processed carrots and spinach in women. *J Nutr* 1998;128:913–916.

Rolls, B., L. Roe, and J. Meengs. Salad and satiety: Energy density and portion size of a first-course salad affect energy intake at lunch. *J Am Diet A* 2004;104:1570–1576.

Sesso, H., J. Buring, E. Norkus, et al. Plasma lycopene, other carotenoids, and retinol and the risk of cardiovascular disease in women. *Am J Clin N* 2004;79:47–53.

Slattery, M., J. Benson, K. Ma, et al. Trans-fatty acids and colon cancer. *Nutr Cancer* 2001;39:170–175.

Stone, K., T. Duong, D. Sellmeyer, et al. Broccoli may be good for bones. *J Bone Min* 1999;14:F272.

Thorogood, M., J. Mann, P. Appleby, et al. Risk of death from cancer and ischemic heart disease in meat and non-meat eaters. *Br Med J* 1994;308:1667–1671.

Tsatsakis, A., I. Tsakiris, M. Tzatzarakis, et al. Three-year study of fenthion and dimethoate pesticides in olive oil from organic and conventional cultivation. *Food Addit Contam* 2003;20:553–559.

Vermunt, S., W. Pasman, G. Schaafsma, et al. Effects of sugar intake on body weight. *Obes Rev* 2003;4:91–99.

Zheng, W., and S. Wang. Oxygen radical absorbing capacity of phenolics in blueberries, cranberries, chokeberries, and lingonberries. *J Agric Food* 2003;51:502–509.

Habit 5

Brownell, K. *Food Fight: The Inside Story of the Food Industry, America's Obesity Crisis, and What We Can Do About It.* New York, Contemporary Books/McGraw-Hill, 2003.

Dulloo, A., C. Duret, D. Rohrer, et al. Efficacy of a green tea extract rich in catechin polyphenols and caffeine in increasing 24-h energy expenditure and fat oxidation in humans. *Am J Clin N* 1999;70:1040–1045.

Heaney, R., M. Davies, and J. Barger-Lux. Calcium and weight: Clinical studies. *J Am Col N* 2002;21:152S–155S.

Painter, J., B. Wansink, et al. How visibility and convenience influence candy consumption. *Appetite* 2002;38(3):237–238.

Rolls, B., E. Bell, and M. Thorwart. Water incorporated into a food but not served with a food decreases energy intake in lean women. *Am J Clin N* 1999;70:448–455.

Rolls, B., I. Fedoroff, J. Guthrie, et al. Foods with different satiating effects in humans. *Appetite* 1990;15:115–126.

Velthuis-te, E., K. Westerterp, and H. van den Berg. Impact of moderately energy-restricted diet on energy metabolism and body composition in non-obese men. *Int J Obes* 1995;19:318–324.

Wansink, B. Environmental factors that increase the food intake and consumption volume of unknowing consumers. *Ann Rev Nutr* 2004;24:455–479.

Wing, R., R. Jeffery, L. Burton, et al. Food provision versus structured meal plans in the behavioral treatment of obesity. *Int J Obes* 1996;20:56–62.

Zemel, M. Regulation of adiposity and obesity risk by dietary calcium: Mechanisms and implications. *J Am Col N* 2002; 21:146S–151S.

Habit 6

Amatruda, J., M. Statt, and S. Welle. Total and resting energy expenditure in obese women reduced to ideal body weight. *J Clin Invest* 1993;92:1236–1242.

Blair, S., and T. Church. The fitness, obesity, and health equation: Is physical activity the common denominator? *J Am Med A* 2004;292:1232–1234.

Brink, P., and K. Ferguson. The decision to lose weight. *W J Nurs R* 1998;20:84–102.

CDC Office of Communications. Obesity costs states billions in medical expenses. January 21, 2004.

Clark, D., F. Tomas, R. Withers, et al. Energy metabolism in free-living, "large-eating" and small-eating women: Studies using H_2O. *Br J Nutr* 1994;72:21–31.

Clark, H., C. Harrison, C. Reid, et al. Effect of supplements of fruit and vegetables on food intake, body weight, and appetite among Scottish consumers. *P Nutr Soc* 2000; Spring:55A.

Eisenberg, M., R. Olson, D. Neumark-Sztainer, et al. Correlations between family meals and psychosocial well-being among adolescents. *Arch Pediatr Adol* 2004;158: 792–796.

Fitzgerald, S., A. Kriska, M. Pereira, et al. Associations among physical activity, television watching, and obesity in adult Pima Indians. *Med Sci Spt* 1997;29:910–915.

Fletcher, A. *Thin for Life: 10 Keys to Success from People Who Have Lost Weight and Kept It Off.* Boston, Houghton Mifflin, 2003.

Foreyt, J., and K. Goodrick. The ultimate triumph of obesity. *Lancet* 1995;346:134–135.

Gore, S., J. Foster, V. DiLillo, et al. Television viewing and snacking. *Eat Behav* 2003;4:399–405.

Gorsky, R., E. Pamuk, D. Williamson, et al. The 25-year health care costs of women who remain overweight after 40 years of age. *Am J Prev Med* 1996;12:388–394.

Hu, F., T. Li, G. Colditz, et al. Television viewing and other sedentary behaviors in relation to risk of obesity and type 2 diabetes mellitus in women. *J Am Med A* 2003;289: 1785–1791.

Klem, M., R. Wing, W. Lang, et al. Does weight-loss maintenance become easier over time? *Obes Res* 2000; 8:438–444.

Klem, M., R.Wing, M. McGuire, et al. A descriptive study of individuals successful at long-term maintenance of substantial weight loss. *Am J Clin N* 1997;66:239–246.

Lavery, M., and J. Loewry. Identifying predictive variables for long-term weight change after participation in a weight-loss program. *J Am Diet A* 1993;93:1017–1024.

McGuire, M., R. Wing, M. Klem, et al. Long-term maintenance of weight loss: Do people who lose weight through various weight-loss methods use different behaviors to maintain their weight? *Int J Obes* 1998;22: 572–577.

McGuire, M., R. Wing, M. Klem, et al. What predicts weight regain in a group of successful weight losers? *J Cons Clin* 1999;67:177–185.

McGuire, M., R. Wing, M. Klem, et al. Behavioral strategies of individuals who have maintained long-term weight losses. *Obes Res* 1999;7:334–341.

Popkin, B., and J. Udry. Adolescent obesity increases significantly in second- and third-generation U.S.

immigrants: The National Longitudinal Study of Adolescent Health. *J Nutr* 1998;128:701–706.

Raynor, H., C. Kilanowski, I. Esterlis, et al. A cost-analysis of adopting a healthful diet in a family-based obesity treatment program. *J Am Diet A* 2002;102:645–656.

St. Jeor, S., R. Brunner, M. Harrington, et al. Who are the weight maintainers? *Obes Res* 1995;3:S249–S259.

Sexton, M., D. Bross, J. Hebel, et al. Risk-factor changes in wives with husbands at high risk of coronary heart disease (CHD): The spin-off effect. *J Behav Med* 1987;10: 251–261.

Shattuck, A., E. White, and A. Kristal. How women's adopted low-fat diets affect their husbands. *Am J Pub He* 1992; 82:1244–1250.

Shick, S., R. Wing, M. Klem, et al. Persons successful at long-term weight loss and maintenance continue to consume a low-energy, low-fat diet. *J Am Diet A* 1998;98:408–413.

Van den Bree, M., L. Eaves, and J. Dwyer. Genetic and environmental influences on eating patterns of twins aged more than or equal to 50 years. *Am J Clin N* 1999;70: 456–465.

Wadden, T., R. Vogt, G. Foster, et al. Exercise and the maintenance of weight loss: One-year follow-up of a controlled clinical trial. *J Cons Clin* 1998;66:429–433.

Weinsier, R., T. Nagy, G. Hunger, et al. Do adaptive changes in metabolic rate favor weight regain in weight-reduced individuals? An examination of the set point theory. *Am J Clin N* 2000;72:1088–1094.

Williams, G., V. Grow, Z. Freedman, et al. Motivational predictors of weight loss and weight-loss maintenance. *J Pers Soc* 1996;70:115–126.

Williamson, D. Dietary intake and physical activity as "predictors" of weight gain in observational, prospective studies of adults. *Nutr Rev* 1996;54:S101–S109.

Wing, R., and J. Hill: Successful weight-loss maintenance. *Ann R Nutr* 2001;21:323–341.

Habit 7

Ainslie, P., I. Campbell, K. Frayn, et al. Energy balance, metabolism, hydration, and performance during strenuous hill walking: The effect of age. *J App Physl* 2002;93: 714–723.

Alpert, J., and M. Fava. Nutrition and depression: The role of folate. *Nutr Rev* 1997;145–149.

Avena, N., and B. Hoebel. Amphetamine-sensitized rats show sugar-induced hyperactivity (cross-sensitization) and sugar hyperphagia. *Phar Bioc Be* 2003;74:635–639.

Berr, C., B. Balansard, J. Arnaud, et al. Cognitive decline is associated with systemic oxidative stress: The EVA study. *J Am Ger So* 2000;48:1285–1291.

Blair, A., V. Lewis, and D. Booth. Does emotional eating interfere with success in attempts at weight control? *Appetite* 1990;15:151–157.

Blundell, J. Nutritional manipulations for altering food intake. *Ann NY Acad* 1987;499:144–155.

Blundell, J., S. Green, and V. Burley. Carbohydrates and human appetite. *Am J Clin N* 1994;59(suppl):728S–734S.

Colantuoni, C., P. Rada, J. McCarthy, et al. Evidence that intermittent, excessive sugar intake causes endogenous opioid dependence. *Obes Res* 2002;10:478–488.

Colantuoni, C., J. Schwenker, J. McCarthy, et al. Excessive sugar intake alters binding to dopamine and opioid receptors in the brain. *Neuroreport* 2001;12:3549–3552.

Cotton, J., V. Burley, J. Weststrate, et al. Dietary fat and appetite: Similarities and differences in the satiating effect of meals supplemented with either fat or carbohydrate. *J Hum Nutr Diet* 1994;7:11–24.

Delarue, J., O. Matzinger, C. Binnert, et al. Fish oil prevents the adrenal activation elicited by mental stress in healthy men. *Diabetes Metab* 2003;29:289–295.

Drewnowski, A., D. Krahn, M. Demitrack, et al. Taste responses and preferences for sweet high-fat foods: Evidence for opioid involvement. *Physl Behav* 1992;51:371–379.

Fava, M., J. Borus, J. Alpert, et al. Folate, vitamin B$_{12}$, and homocysteine and major depressive disorder. *Am J Psychiat* 1997;154:426–428.

Feunekes, G., C. deGraaf, and W. vanStaveren. Social facilitation of food intake is mediated by meal duration. *Physl Behav* 1995;58:551–558.

Hammersley, R., and M. Reid. Are simple carbohydrates physiologically addictive? *Addict Res* 1997;5:145–160.

Hasing, L., A. Wahlin, B. Winblad, et al. Further evidence on the effects of vitamin B$_{12}$ and folate levels on episodic memory functioning: A population-based study of healthy very old adults. *Biol Psych* 1999;45:1472–1480.

Helm, K., P. Rada, and B. Hoebel. Cholecystokinin combined with serotonin in the hypothalamus limits accumbens dopamine release while increasing acetylcholine: A possible satiation mechanism. *Brain Res* 2003;963:290–297.

Hetherington, M., and J. Macdiarmid. Pleasure and excess: Liking for and overconsumption of chocolate. *Physl Behav* 1995;57:27–35.

Hibbeln, J. Fish consumption and major depression. *Lancet* 1998;351:1213.

Hibbeln, J., M. Linnoila, J. Umhau, et al. Essential fatty acids predict metabolites of serotonin and dopamine in cerebrospinal fluid among healthy control subjects, and early- and late-onset alcoholics. *Biol Psychi* 1998;44:235–242.

Hoebel, B., C. Colantuoni, J. Schwenker, et al. Sugar dependence: Neural and behavioral signs of sensitization and withdrawal. *Am J Clin N* 2002;75:241.

Howarth, N., E. Saltzman, and S. Roberts. Dietary fiber and weight regulation. *Nutr Rev* 2001;59:129–139.

Joseph, J., B. Shukitt-Hale, N. Denisova, et al. Reversals of age-related declines in neuronal signal transduction, cognitive, and motor behavioral deficits with blueberry, spinach, or strawberry dietary supplementation. *J Neurosc* 1999;19:8114–8121.

J Am Diet A 1996;96:1253. Study finds men and women overeat for different reasons.

Kleiner, S. Water: An essential nutrient. *Am J Diet A* 1999; 99:200–206.

Kromhout, D., B. Boemberg, J. Seidell, et al. Physical activity and dietary fiber determine population body fat levels: The Seven Countries Study. *Int J Obes* 2001;25:301–306.

Mamalakis, G., M. Kiriakakis, G. Tsibinos, et al. Depression and adipose polyunsaturated fatty acids in the survivors of the seven countries study population of Crete. *Prost Leuk* 2004;70:495–501.

Martin, A., K. Youdim, A. Szprengiel, et al. Roles of vitamins E and C on neurodegenerative diseases and cognitive performance. *Nutr Rev* 2002;60:308–326.

Meguid, M., S. Fetissov, M. Varma, et al. Hypothalamic dopamine and serotonin in the regulation of food intake. *Nutrition* 2000;16:843–857.

Metzner, H., D. Lamphiear, N. Wheeler, et al. Relationship between frequency of eating and adiposity in adult men and women in the Tecumseh Community Health Study. *Am J Clin N* 1977;30:712–715.

Nilsson, K., L. Gustafson, and B. Hultberg. Improvement of cognitive functions after cobalamine/folate supplementation in elderly patients with dementia and elevated plasma homocysteine. *Int J Ger Psy* 2001;16: 609–614.

Pelchat, M. Of human bondage: Food craving, obsession, compulsion, and addiction. *Physl Behav* 2002;76: 347–352.

Putnam, J., J. Allshouse, and L. Kantor. U.S. per capita food supply trends: More calories, refined carbohydrates, and fats. *Food Rev* 2002;25:2–15.

Roberts, S. High-glycemic index foods, hunger, and obesity. Is there a connection? *Nutr Rev* 2000;58:163–169.

Rogers, P., A. Kainth, and H. Smit. A drink of water can improve or impair mental performance depending on small differences in thirst. *Appetite* 2001;36:57–58.

Stubbs, R. Macronutrient effects on appetite. *Int J Obes* 1995; 19:S11–S19.

Tanskanen, A., J. Hibbeln, J. Tuomilehto, et al. Fish consumption and depressive symptoms in the general population of Finland. *Psych Serv* 2001;52:529–531.

Vandewater, K., and Z. Vickers. Higher-protein foods produce greater sensory-specific satiety. *Physl Behav* 1996;59: 579–583.

Warwick, Z., W. Hall, T. Pappas, et al. Taste and smell sensations enhance the satiating effect of both a high-carbohydrate and a high-fat meal in humans. *Physl Behav* 1993;53:553–563.

Zador, D., P. Wall, and I. Webster. High sugar intake in a group of women on methadone maintenance in South Western Sydney, Australia. *Addiction* 1996;97:1053–1061.

Habit 8

Alper, C., and R. Mattes. Effects of chronic peanut consumption on energy balance and hedonics. *Int J Obes* 2002;26:1129–1137.

Astrup, A. Carbohydrate and obesity. *Int J Obes* 1995;19: S27–S37.

Baba, N., R. Sultan, N. Cortas, et al. Diet composition affects weight gain, adiposity, and blood parameters in healthy human volunteers. *Nutr Res* 1999;19:1313–1326.

Ball, K., W. Brown, and D. Crawford. Who does not gain weight? Prevalence and predictors of weight maintenance in young women. *Int J Obes* 2002;26:1570–1578.

Barkeling, B., S. Rossner, and H. Bjorvell. Effects of a high-protein meal (meat) and a high-carbohydrate meal (vegetarian) on satiety measured by automated computerized monitoring of subsequent food intake, motivation to eat, and food preferences. *Int J Obes* 1990;14:743–751.

Blackburn, G., B. Kanders, P. Lavin, et al. The effect of aspartame as part of a multidisciplinary weight-control program on short- and long-term control of body weight. *Am J Clin N* 1997;65:409–418.

Champagne, C., N. Baker, J. DeLany, et al. Assessment of energy intake underreporting by doubly labeled water and observations on reported nutrient intakes in children. *J Am Diet A* 1998;98:426–430.

Fedoroff, I., J. Polivy, and C. Herman. The effect of pre-exposure to food cues on the eating behavior of restrained and unrestrained eaters. *Appetite* 1997;28:33–47.

Fischer, M., and P. LaChance. Nutrition evaluation of published weight-reducing diets. *J Am Diet A* 1985;85: 450–454.

Foster, G., H. Wyatt, J. Hill, et al. A randomized trial for a low-carbohydrate diet for obesity. *N Eng J Med* 2003;348: 2082–2090.

Golay, A., A. Allaz, J. Ybarra, et al. Similar weight loss with low-energy food-combining or balanced diets. *Int J Obes* 2000;24:492–496.

Gorin, A., S. Phelan, R. Wing, et al. Promoting long-term weight-loss control: Does dieting consistency matter? *Int J Obes* 2004;28:278–282.

Hensrud, D., R. Weisnier, B. Darnell, et al. A prospective study of weight maintenance in obese subjects reduced to normal body weight without weight-loss training. *Am J Clin N* 1994;60:688–694.

Horton, T., H. Drougas, A. Brachey, et al. Fat and carbohydrate overfeeding in humans: Different effects on energy storage. *Am J Clin N* 1995;62:19–29.

Howarth, N., E. Saltzman, and S. Roberts. Dietary fiber and weight regulation. *Nutr Rev* 2001;59:129–139.

Kajioka, T., S. Tsuzuku, H. Shimokata, et al. Effects of intentional weight cycling on nonobese young women. *Metabolism* 2002;51:149–154.

Kennedy, E., S. Bowman, J. Spence, et al. Popular diets: Correlation to health, nutrition, and obesity. *J Am Diet A* 2001;101:411–420.

Kirk, S., and A. Hill. Exploring the food beliefs and eating behavior of successful and unsuccessful dieters. *J Hum Nutr Diet* 1997;10:331–341.

Kromhout, D., B. Boemberg, J. Seidell, et al. Physical activity and dietary fiber determine population body fat levels: The Seven Countries Study. *Int J Obes* 2001;25:301–306.

Kruger, J., D. Galuska, M. Serdula, et al. Attempting to lose weight: Specific practices among U.S. adults. *Am J Prev Med* 2004;26:402–406.

Lacey, J., A. Tershakovec, and G. Foster. Acupuncture for the treatment of obesity: A review of the evidence. *Int J Obes* 2003;27:419–427.

Latner, J., and M. Schwartz. The effects of a high-carbohydrate, high-protein, or balanced lunch upon later food intake and hunger ratings. *Appetite* 1999;33:119–128.

Lavin, P., P. Sanders, M. Mackey, et al. Intense sweeteners use and weight change among women: A critique of the Stellman and Garfinkel study. *J Am Col N* 1994;13:102–105.

Mertz, W., J. Tsui, J. Judd, et al. What are people really eating? The relation between energy intake derived from estimated diet records and intake determined to maintain body weight. *Am J Clin N* 1991;54:291–295.

The National Heart, Lung, and Blood Institute Expert Panel on the Identification, Evaluation, and Treatment of Overweight and Obesity in Adults: Executive summary of the clinical guidelines on the identification, evaluation, and treatment of overweight and obesity in adults. *J Am Diet A* 1998;98:1178–1191.

Olson, M., S. Kelsey, V. Bittner, et al. Weight cycling and high-density lipoprotein cholesterol in women: Evidence of an adverse effect. *J Am Col C* 2000;36:1565–1571.

Pasman, W., M. Westerterp-Plantenga, and W. Saris. The effectiveness of long-term supplementation of carbohydrate, chromium, fiber, and caffeine on weight maintenance. *Int J Obes* 1997;21:1143–1151.

Polivy, J. Psychological consequences of food restriction. *J Am Diet A* 1996;96:589–592.

Raben, A., L. Agerholm-Larsen, A. Flint, et al. Meals with similar energy densities but rich in protein, fat, carbohydrate, or alcohol have different effects on energy expenditure and substrate metabolism but not on appetite and energy intake. *Am J Clin N* 2003;77:91–100.

Roberts, D. Quick weight loss: Sorting fad from fact. *Med J Aust* 2001;175:637–640.

Roberts, S. High-glycemic index foods, hunger, and obesity. Is there a connection? *Nutr Rev* 2000;58:163–169.

Seidell, J. Dietary fat and obesity: An epidemiologic perspective. *Am J Clin N* 1998;67:S546–S550.

Shide, D., and B. Rolls. Information about the fat content of preloads influences energy intake in healthy women. *J Am Diet A* 1995;95:993–998.

Singh, R., M. Niaz, and S. Ghosh. Effect on central obesity and associated disturbances of low-energy, fruit- and vegetable-enriched prudent diet in North Indians. *Postgrad Med J* 1994;70:895–900.

Speechly, D., and R. Buffenstein. Greater appetite control associated with an increased frequency of eating in lean males. *Appetite* 1999;33:285–297.

Strauss, J., A. Doyle, and R. Kreipe. The paradoxical effect of diet commercials on reinhibition of dietary restraint. *Abn Psych* 1994;103:441–444.

Stubbs, R. Macronutrient effects on appetite. *Int J Obes* 1995; 19(S5):11S–19S.

Taylor, M., and J. Garrow. Compared with nibbling, neither gorging nor a morning fast affect short-term energy balance in obese patients in a chamber calorimeter. *Int J Obes* 2001;25:519–528.

Tucker, L., and M. Kano. Dietary fat and body fat: A multivariate study of 205 adult females. *Am J Clin N* 1992;56:616–622.

Urbszat, D., P. Herman, and J. Polivy. Eat, drink, and be merry, for tomorrow we diet. *J Abn Psych* 2002;111:396–401.

Vandewater, K., and Z. Vickers. Higher-protein foods produce greater sensory-specific satiety. *Physl Behav* 1996;59: 579–583.

Weiss, D. How to help your patients lose weight: Current therapy for obesity. *Clev Clin J* 2000;67:739–753.

Westerterp, K., S. Wilson, and V. Rolland. Diet induced thermogenesis measured over 24-h in a respiration chamber: Effect of diet composition. *Int J Obes* 1999;23: 287–292.

Westerterp-Plantenga, M., E. Kovacs, and K. Melanson. Habitual meal frequency and energy intake regulation in partially temporally isolated men. *Int J Obes* 2002;26: 102–110.

Westerterp-Plantenga, M., V. Rolland, S. Wilson, et al. Satiety related to 24-hour diet-induced thermogenesis during high-protein/carbohydrate versus high-fat diets measured in a respiration chamber. *Eur J Clin N* 1999;53:495–502.

Wyatt, H., O. Grunwald, C. Mosca, et al. Long-term weight loss and breakfast in subjects in the National Weight Control Registry. *Obes Res* 2002;10:78–82.

Habit 9

Breslow, R., and B. Smothers. Drinking patterns and body mass index in never smokers. *Am J Epidem* 2005;161:368–376.

Buemann, B., S. Toubro, and A. Astrup. The effect of wine or beer versus a carbonated soft drink, served at a meal, on ad libitum energy intake. *Int J Obes* 2002;26:1367–1372.

De Groot, L., and P. Zock. Moderate alcohol intake and mortality. *Nutr Rev* 1998;56:25–26.

DiMeglio, D., and R. Mattes. Liquid versus solid carbohydrate: Effects on food intake and body weight. *Int J Obes* 2000; 24:794–800.

Elliott, S., N. Keim, J. Stern, et al. Fructose, weight gain, and the insulin resistance syndrome. *Am J Clin N* 2002;76: 911–922.

Frankel, E., J. Kanner, J. German, et al. Inhibition of oxidation of human low-density lipoprotein by phenolic substances in red wine. *Lancet* 1993;341:454–457.

Goldberg, I., L. Mosca, M. Piano, et al. Wine and your heart. *Stroke* 2001;32:591–594.

Gronbaek, M., U. Becker, D. Johansen, et al. Type of alcohol consumed and mortality from all causes, coronary heart disease, and cancer. *Ann Int Med* 2000;133:411–419.

Guo, X., B. Warden, S. Paeratakul, et al. Healthy eating index and obesity. *Eur J Clin N* 2004;May 19.

Guthrie, J., and J. Morton. Sources of added calories in the diets of Americans. *FASEB J* 1999;13:A695.

Halkjaer, J., T. Sorensen, A. Tjonneland, et al. Food and drinking patterns as predictors of six-year BMI-adjusted changes in waist circumference. *Br J Nutr* 2004;92: 735–748.

Halsted, C., J. Villanueva, A. Devlin, et al. Metabolic interactions of alcohol and folate. *J Nutr* 2002;132: 2367–2372.

Hetherington, M., F. Cameron, D. Wallis, et al. Stimulation of appetite by alcohol. *Physl Behav* 2001;74:283–289.

Lands, W. Alcohol, calories, and appetite. *Vitam Horm* 1998; 54:31–49.

Ludwig, D., K. Peterson, and S. Gortmaker. Relation between consumption of sugar-sweetened drinks and childhood obesity. *Lancet* 2001;357:505–508.

Mattes, R., and D. Rothacker. Beverage viscosity is inversely related to postprandial hunger in humans. *Physl Behav* 2001;74:551–557.

Rolls, B., E. Bell, and M. Thorwart. Water incorporated into a food but not served with a food decreases energy intake in lean women. *Am J Clin N* 1999;70:448–455.

Sato, M., N. Maulik, and D. Das. Cardioprotection with alcohol. *Ann NY Acad* 2002;957:122–135.

Schulze, M., J. Manson, D. Ludwig, et al. Sugar-sweetened beverages, weight gain, and incidence of type 2 diabetes in

young and middle-aged women. *J Am Med A* 2004;
292:927–934.

Soleas, G., E. Diamandis, and D. Goldberg. Wine as a
biological fluid: History, production, and role in disease
prevention. *J Cl Lab An* 1997;11:287–313.

Urgano-Marquez, A., R. Estruch, J. Fernandez-Sola, et al. The
greater risk of alcoholic cardiomyopathy and myopathy in
women compared with men. *J Am Med A* 1995;274:
149–154.

Wannamethee, S., A. Field, G. Colditz, et al. Alcohol intake
and eight-year weight gain in women. *Obes Res* 2004;12:
1386–1396.

Habit 10

Abernathy, R., and D. Black. Healthy body weights: An
alternative perspective. *Am J Clin N* 1996;63:S448–S451.

Davidhizar, R., and R. Shearer. Increasing self-confidence
through self-talk. *Home Healthc Nurse* 1996;14:119–122.

Meisler, J., and S. St. Jeor. American Health Foundation Round
Table on Healthy Weight. *Am J Clin N* 1996;63:S409–
S411.

———. Summary and recommendations from the American
Health Foundation Expert Panel on Healthy Weight. *Am
J Clin N* 1996;63:474S–477S.

Murray, M. Coping with change: Self-talk. *Hosp Pract* 2000;
35:118–120.

Peden, A., L. Hall, M. Rayens, et al. Reducing negative
thinking and depressive symptoms in college women. *J
Nurs Scholarsh* 2000;32:145–151.

Schneider, J. Relations among self-talk, self-consciousness, and
self-knowledge. *Psychol Rep* 2002;91:807–812.

Simple Steps, Big Results

Gorin, A., S. Phelan, R. Wing, et al. Promoting long-term weight control: Does dieting consistency matter? *Int J Obes* 2004;28:278–281.

Kayman, S., W. Bruvold, and J. Stern. Maintenance and relapse after weight loss in women. *Am J Clin N* 1990;52: 800–807.

Kirkland, L., and R. Anderson. Achieving healthy weights. *Can Fam Phys* 1993;39:157–158, 161–162.

Mattes, R. Soup and satiety. *Physl Behav* 2005;83:739–747.

Index

Abramson, Edward, 52–53, 54, 55
Activity/exercise logs, 154, 158
Aging, 104, 155, 250
Alcohol, 94, 140, 166, 170, 190, 220–31, 241, 264
  annual consumption of, 221–22
  benefits of, 222–24
  dark side of, 224–26
  managing key situations, 230–31
  nutrition and, 228–29
  spillover effect of, 221–22
  ten rules for drinking, 229
All-or-nothing approach, 235–52
  reasons for failure of, 236–37
  weight and, 237–38
Antecedent (of overeating), 207–9
Antioxidants, 104, 105, 112, 113, 173, 222, 223, 228
Arthritis, 198
Asthma, 113
Atherosclerosis, 223

Babies and weight gain, 56, 155
Baranowski, Tom, 153
Bazzano, Lydia, 6
Beano, 155
Beans, 6, 16–18, 84, 154–55, 264
Beer, 220, 224
Behavior (overeating), 207–9
Behavior Therapy (journal), 171
Berries, 112
Beverages, 114, 217–34. *See also* specific beverages
Birth defects, 110, 225
Block, Gladys, 101–2
Blood clots, 105, 222, 224
Blood sugar, 6, 178, 210
Blumberg, Jeffrey, 6, 102, 110–11, 116
Body, listening to, 180
Body mass index (BMI), 208, 240
Bravata, Dena M., 199
Bray, George, 114, 199
Breakfast, 15, 46–47, 169–70, 187, 210, 263
  guidelines for, 17, 48–49, 212
  mindful, 36–40
  weight control and, 37–38

Breakfast log, 38–39
Brownell, Kelly, 51–52, 134, 191, 196, 200, 201, 209

Caffeine, 170, 171–73, 174, 188, 189–90
Calcium, 6, 7, 8, 16, 17, 110, 115, 131, 154, 177, 225
Callaway, Wayne C., 46, 187, 237
Calories
  in alcohol, 220
  in beverages, 217–20, 263
  counting, 205–6
  cutting 100 per day, 264
  daily increase in, 2, 5, 115, 186
  decrease required for weight loss, 200, 205–6
  diet of 1,200–2,000, 90–91
  exercise and, 94, 96, 156
  fast food impact on intake, 4
  in fat, 209
  gender differences in need for, 54
  in a healthy diet, 213
  inadequate intake of, 177, 200
  invisible, 26–29, 45
  quick guide to tracking, 207
  in snacks, 32
  underestimation of intake, 78
Cancer, 7, 37, 80
  alcohol intake and, 223, 224, 225–26, 227, 228–29
  breast, 34, 105, 225–26, 227, 228–29, 237, 240
  cervical, 103
  colon, 6, 8, 34, 103, 115, 131, 154
  dietary fat and, 3, 115
  esophageal, 103, 225
  liver, 103
  lung, 103
  mouth, 225
  non-Hodgkin's lymphoma, 104
  pancreatic, 103
  produce intake and, 102, 103, 104, 105, 110, 111, 112, 113, 116
  stomach, 103
  throat, 225
  visceral fat and, 175, 240

Carbohydrates, 197, 209, 220. *See also* Low-carbohydrate diets
  in breakfast, 46–47
  mood and, 170, 171, 175, 181, 186, 188
  quality, 184–85, 210–11
Carotenoids, 105, 111
Cartland, Barbara, 254
Cataracts, 102, 110
Cellulite, 240
Children, 28, 56–57, 66, 135–36, 165–66. *See also* Families
Cholesterol levels, 6, 33, 94, 103, 163–65. *See also* HDL-cholesterol; LDL-cholesterol
Christensen, Larry, 173, 174
Clark, Nancy, 232
Consequences (of overeating), 207–9
Consistent eating patterns, 46
Cooper, Kenneth, 94
Cortisol, 31–33, 175
Craig, Winston, 116–17
Cravings, working with, 171
Cruciferous vegetables, 103

Dallman, Mary, 174, 180
Dark green leafy vegetables, 110–11
Dehydration, 187, 232–33
Dementia, 155, 222, 223, 225
Depression, 37, 166, 190
  alcohol intake and, 225
  caffeine and, 171–73
  omega-3 fats and, 155, 172, 198
  sugar and, 174, 188
Desserts, 262–63, 265
Diabetes, 6, 7, 80, 157, 210, 213, 240
  exercise and, 250
  moderate weight loss and, 237
  produce intake and, 102, 104, 105
  snacking and, 34
  visceral fat and, 175
Diet foods, 202. *See also* Fat-free foods
Diets. *See also* Quick-fix diets
  annual expenditures on products, 192
  example of healthy, 212–13
  keeping perspective on, 71–73
  very-low-calorie, 205
  weight gain caused by, 176–78
Dinners
  example of healthy, 17, 213
  ten-minute, 160–61
Dishonesty, 75–99
  consequences of, 81–82
  about exercise, 76, 80–81

about portion size, 82–87
  reasons for, 78–81
Donkersloot, Mary, 66, 69
Drewnowski, Adam, 93, 94, 106, 181
Druck, Ken, 65–66, 67

Eating disorders, 194
Eckel, Robert H., 152, 153, 197
Edelstein, Sharon, 31
Endorphins, 168, 171, 176
Estrogen, 225, 241
Excuses, 149–66
Exercise, 152, 205, 211–12, 214, 240
  all-or-nothing approach to, 249–51
  aerobic, 251
  determining adequacy of, 94–96
  excuses for avoiding, 154, 155, 156–57, 163–65
  getting started, 158
  inaccurate estimates of, 76, 80–81, 156
  mood and, 170, 190
  obtaining physician approval for, 95
  overeating and, 156, 263
  planning for, 132
  simple steps for increasing, 261, 262
  warming up and cooling down, 251

Families, 57–58, 65–70, 165–66
Fast food, 3–4, 15, 59, 85, 92–93, 161, 162, 210, 266
Fat (body). *See also* Body mass index
  alcohol and, 221, 224
  dietary fat stored as, 197, 209
  visceral/intra-abdominal, 33, 175, 240–41
Fat (dietary)
  in cheese, 8
  cutting out all, 197–98
  decreasing intake of, 209–11
  estimating portion size, 84–85
  food labels on, 94, 262
  increased intake of, 3, 115
  monounsaturated, 7
  mood and, 175
  omega-3, 18, 155, 172, 198
  recommended intake of, 18, 88
  satiety quotient of, 187, 197, 220
  saturated, 6, 8, 198
  trans, 115, 198
Fat-free foods, 93, 262–63
Fatigue, 37, 38, 40, 170, 171, 232, 233
Favorite foods, 67, 69–70, 213–15

Fiber, 6, 7, 47, 104–5, 110, 111, 112, 113, 186, 210
Fibroid tumors, 113
Fish, 15, 17, 18, 155, 177
Fit Fat After Forty (Peeke), 241
Fit for Life diet, 195
5-a-Day for Better Health program, 106, 162
Flavonoids, 105, 112, 222
Flavor, 69, 187
Fletcher, Anne, 9, 10, 12, 14, 15, 41, 133, 150, 151, 161, 195, 210, 213, 236
Food allergies, 8, 154
Food combining, 196–97
Food diaries, 37, 40–42, 75–76, 89–91, 127–29, 132, 133, 204, 205–6, 208
    creating solutions from, 45–46
    different-colored ink for, 76, 89
    mood recorded in, 178, 179
    reviewing, 43
Food Fight (Brownell), 134
Food Guide Pyramid, 2, 3
Foreyt, John, 2, 11, 14, 79, 89, 152, 156, 169, 180, 196, 197, 200, 201, 206, 208, 250–51
Free radicals, 104, 105, 173, 223, 224, 228
Fruit-flavored drinks, 114
Fruits and vegetables. *See* Produce

Gallstones, 205
Genetic factors in weight, 152, 153
Glucose, 36, 40, 171, 188, 199
Glycemic index, 6, 210
Glycogen, 199
Goals, 96–97, 158
    life, 267
    realistic, 66, 214
    ultimate, 261–66
Golden-colored vegetables, 111–12
Goldin, Barry, 8
Grains, 3, 6, 83. *See also* Whole grains
    quality, 184–85
    recommended intake of, 16, 17, 88
Grazing, 181. *See also* Snacking/nibbling
Green tea, 131
Grocery shopping, 137, 140, 141–45, 265

Hair loss, 205
Hangovers, 231
HDL-cholesterol, 103, 203, 222
Health
    commitment to, 215–16
    eating for, 14–15

focus on, 181, 264
size and, 240–41
Healthy-Habits Pyramid, 257, 259–61
Heart attack, 165, 222
Heart disease, 6, 7, 8, 37, 80, 154, 205, 213
    alcohol intake and, 223, 224, 226
    dietary fat and, 3, 115, 198
    exercise and, 250
    fish and, 155
    moderate weight loss and, 237, 238
    produce intake and, 102, 103, 104, 105, 110, 112, 113, 116
    snacking and, 34
    visceral fat and, 175, 240
    yo-yo dieting and, 203
Hibbeln, Joseph, 172
High-fructose corn syrup (HFCS), 188, 218–19
High-protein diets, 200
Hill, Gretchen, 37
Hill, Jim, 9, 10, 95, 96, 128, 134, 136, 211, 212
Hoebel, Bartley, 175
Homocysteine, 103, 172
Hormone replacement therapy, 225
Hunger, 167–68
    dieting and, 176–78, 194–95
    getting in touch with, 178–81
    stomach *vs.* mouth, 180
    stomach *vs.* social, 60
    thirst confused with, 232, 262
Husbands, 52–56, 65–66, 166
Hypertension, 6, 37, 80, 94, 163–65, 213
    exercise and, 250
    moderate weight loss and, 237
    produce intake and, 102, 103, 104
    visceral fat and, 175, 240
    yo-yo dieting and, 203

Immune system, 104
Insulin, 33–34, 210
Iron, 6, 7, 110, 111, 118, 154, 177, 187

Jenkins, David, 33–34
Juice, 16, 118

Kem, Omer, 156
Kesten, Deborah, 47–49
Keys, Ancel, 194
Kidney stones, 232

Kitchen
  cleaning out, 265
  mindless eating in, 27, 45
  revamping, 146–47
  stocking, 67, 135–36
Kiwifruits, 112–13
Kleiner, Susan, 232

Labels, reading, 94, 188–89, 262
Lactobacillus acidophilus, 8
Lactose intolerance, 8, 154
LDL-cholesterol, 33, 103, 222–23, 224
Legumes, 6, 15, 16–18, 88, 177, 210
Lipoprotein lipase (LPL), 152
Low-carbohydrate diets, 3, 93, 109, 198–99
Lunch, example of healthy, 17, 213
Lutein, 105, 110–11
Lycopene, 105, 113–14

Macular degeneration, 110, 223
Magnesium, 6, 7, 110, 113, 118, 225
Mangoes, 112–13
Mattes, Richard, 30, 42–43, 44
McDonald's, 59, 85, 86, 116, 201
McManus, Kathy, 7
Meals
  makeovers for, 68
  maximizing options, 159
  portable, 134–35, 263
  preparing extra, 158
  preparing in quantity, 159
  quick-fix, 159
  readily available, 157
Meat, 8, 15, 17, 84, 87, 88, 177
Memory problems, 37, 40, 47, 80, 110, 172, 173, 198, 225
Menopause, 171, 225, 241
Metabolism, 37, 77, 81, 95, 152, 153, 157, 203
Milk and milk products, 8, 15, 84, 131, 266
  allergies to, 154
  recommended intake of, 16, 88, 177
Mindful eating, 47–49, 60, 180–81
Mindless eating, 25–49, 257
  likely venues for, 27–29
  subconscious rationalizations for, 29
Moderation, 215, 223, 226, 233–34
Mood, 12, 157, 167–90
  breakfast and, 46–47, 169–70, 187
  food relationship with, 170–71
  foods to boost, 172–73, 181–90

handling without food, 205
non-dietary factors in, 190
six food rules to manage, 188–89
Moores, Susan, 26, 27, 30, 31, 44, 45, 57, 89, 117, 118, 135, 163, 190, 213, 226, 243
Motivation, 164
Movies, eating during, 29, 129–30, 168
Mullegan, Hugh, 266
Munter, Carol, 176, 178, 180, 181, 194
Muscle, maintaining, 95, 250

Needs, 51–73
  communicating, 62–63
  setting an example and, 63
  setting limits and, 60–61
Neuropeptide Y (NPY), 37, 171, 187
Neurotransmitters, 187
Night-eating syndrome, 37
Nistico, Vince, 151
Nurses' Health Study, 225
Nutritiondata, 206
Nuts, 7, 15, 18, 88, 131

Oats, 185
Obesity, 94, 102
Oils, 18
Omega-3 fats, 18, 155, 172, 198
100/100 plan, 206
Osteoporosis, 7, 104, 154, 155, 198, 222, 225

Packaged foods, 92–93
Pedometers, 96, 212, 263
Peeke, Pamela, 33, 175, 241
Perfectionism, losing, 11, 212–13
Phelan, Suzanne, 11, 13, 14, 95, 136, 150–51, 161, 209
Phytochemicals, 6, 105, 111, 112, 154, 173
Planning, 125–47
  food diaries in, 128–29, 132, 133
  must-have habits in, 134–36
  realistic, 129–33
  strategies, tactics, and tricks, 138–40
Ponichtera, Brenda, 67
Portion size, 67, 82–87, 117, 214, 263
Potassium, 7, 110, 111, 112, 113, 198, 225
Potatoes, 115–16
Practice, 11, 136, 204–5
Premenstrual syndrome (PMS), 150, 170, 171
Preplanning steps, 8–14
Price of food, 106–7, 161–62
Processed foods, 33

Produce, 32, 101–24, 210
  to avoid, 114–16
  best choices, 110–14
  a dozen ways to eat more, 123
  excuses for skimping on, 106–7
  fifty ways to love, 119–21
  health benefits of, 103–4
  healthful ingredients in, 104–5
  inadequate intake of, 4–5, 105–6
  organic, 122
  poor choices in, 107–10
  portion size, 83, 117
  recommended intake of, 15–16, 17, 88,
    116–17, 177
  simple steps for increasing intake of, 261,
    265
Protein, 7, 8, 46–47, 197, 200, 209, 220
Putnam, Judith, 2, 8, 18, 112–13, 115, 116

Quick-fix diets, 191–216
  debunking of myths, 196–203
  reasons for failure of, 193–96
  spotting gimmicks, 192
Quinoa, 185
Quizzes
  "Am I Sabotaging Myself?" 64–65
  "Are You Getting Enough?" 108–9
  "Can You Tell a Muffin From a Cake?"
    83–85
  "Do You Drink Too Much?" 227
  "How Does Your Diet Rate, Habitwise?"
    20–23
  "Is Now the Right Time for a Change?"
    258

Raffinose, 154
Relapses, 214, 241–43
Responsibility, taking, 166, 253
Restaurant dining, 54, 58–59
  mindless eating during, 27–28
  planning ahead for, 140
  portion size and, 82
  serving solutions for, 70–71
  setting limits during, 61
  simple steps for, 262, 265
Resveratrol, 222, 223
Rewarding oneself, 10–11, 158, 164
Roberts, Susan, 200, 203
Rolls, Barbara, 45, 70, 82, 88, 162, 167, 221,
    228
Rozin, Paul, 87, 92

Sabotage, 54–55, 58, 62, 63–65, 127, 151,
    253
Salad, 131, 201–2
Salad dressing, 18, 59, 116, 201, 266
Salami Principle, 256–61
Salmon, 16, 18, 198
Samuel-Hodge, Carmen D., 79
Self-talk, 238–39, 243–49
Serotonin, 168, 170–71, 172–73, 186, 188
Sesso, Howard D., 113
Set point theory, 153
Skin protection, 111, 116
Skipping meals, 46, 201, 262. See also Breakfast
Sleep, 134, 170, 225, 263
Slips, handling, 214, 241–43
Slow foods, 259–61
Smoking, 190, 223, 241
Snacking/nibbling, 190, 201
    advantages of, 31–36
    healthy foods for, 17, 34–35, 177, 212, 213
    norms for, 32–33
Sobal, Jeffrey, 53
Social pressure, 57–58, 61
Social support system, 170, 190
Soft drinks, 19, 189, 202, 218–20, 226
Soy milk, 7, 15, 16, 84, 131, 154
Stealth nutrition, 118
Stoner, Gary, 112
Strength training, 95, 251
Stress, 12, 31–33, 169, 174–75, 241
Stroke, 6, 104, 105, 165, 222
Subar, Amy, 9, 77
Success, measuring, 12–13, 204
Sugar, 150, 170, 173–76, 218, 219
    addiction to, 175–76
    average annual intake of, 2–3
    recommendations on intake of, 18–19,
      188–89
    rush from, 173–75
Sunlight and mood, 170–71
Sweet potatoes, 115–16, 210

Television, 29, 154, 157, 159, 212, 262
Thought stopping, 139, 246
Time management, 154, 157–59, 160–61, 256
Tomato sauce, 113–14
Toxic environment, 51–52, 134
Tribole, Evelyn, 67–68, 69
Trigger foods, 135, 139, 257

Urinary-tract infections, 104, 232

Vegetables and fruits. *See* Produce
Vegetarians, 103
Visualization, 163, 164
Vitamin supplements, 187, 189, 205, 211,
    228, 264
Vitamins
    A, 113, 118, 225
    B, 7, 8, 110, 118, 154, 198, 233
    B_1, 225
    B_2, 115
    B_6, 187, 188, 225, 228
    B_{12}, 187, 225
    beta-carotene, 104, 105, 111, 116
    C, 103, 104, 107, 110, 111, 112, 113, 115,
        225, 228
    D, 7, 154
    E, 7, 228
    folic acid, 6, 7, 110, 118, 172–73, 187, 189,
        225, 228–29
    K, 110

Wadden, Thomas, 180
Walking, 95, 211
Wansink, Brian, 29, 87, 88–89, 92, 132–33,
    168

Water, 187–88, 219–20, 231–33, 262, 264
Water weight/fluid retention, 77, 199
Waterhouse, Debra, 26, 41, 44–45, 118, 122,
    170, 171
Watson, Ronald, 111
Weighing and measuring food, 89–92
Weight loss
    ABCs of, 206–9
    gradual, 205
    impact of moderate, 237–38
    in a nutshell, 214–15
    rapid, 200–201
Wheat, 184
Wheat germ, 7, 16
Whole grains, 6, 15, 16, 17, 186, 188–89, 199,
    210
Willett, Walter, 104
Willpower, 162–63, 206
Wine, 222–24, 227–29, 230–31, 233–34

Yo-yo dieting, 203
Yogurt, 7, 8, 16, 177
Young, Lisa, 82, 85, 91, 93

Zinc, 6, 7, 154, 225